500 Formulas for AROMATHERAPY

D0479844

500 Formulas for AROMATHERAPY

Mixing Essential Oils for Every Use

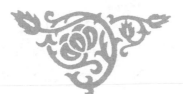

Carol Schiller
& David Schiller

STERLING PUBLISHING CO., INC.
NEW YORK

Library of Congress Cataloging-in-Publication Data

Schiller, Carol.
    500 Formulas for aromatherapy : mixing essential oils for every
use / Carol Schiller and David Schiller.
      p.   cm.
    Includes bibliographical references and indexes.
    ISBN 0-8069-0584-0
    1. Aromatherapy. I. Schiller, David. II. Title. III. Title: Five
hundred formulas for aromatherapy.
RM666.A68S35   1994
615'.321--dc20   93-39895
                                                     CIP

34   36   38   37   35   33

Published in 1994 by Sterling Publishing Co., Inc.
387 Park Avenue South, New York, NY 10016
© 1994 by Carol Schiller and David Schiller
Distributed in Canada by Sterling Publishing
ᶜ/ₒ Canadian Manda Group, 165 Dufferin Street,
Toronto, Ontario, Canada M6K 3H6
Distributed in Great Britain by Chrysalis Books Group PLC
The Chrysalis Building, Bramley Road, London W10 6SP, England
Distributed in Australia by Capricorn Link (Australia) Pty. Ltd.
P.O. Box 704, Windsor, NSW 2756, Australia

Manufactured in the United States of America
All rights reserved

Sterling ISBN-13: 978-0-8069-0584-6
ISBN-10: 0-8069-0584-0

For information about custom editions, special sales, premium and
corporate purchases, please contact Sterling Special Sales
Department at 800-805-5489 or specialsales@sterlingpub.com.

Before using any formulas in the book, please read the Safety Guidelines very carfeully. The essential oils are very potent substances and **MUST** *be handled with care. Their safe and proper use is the sole responsibility of the persons(s) using any of the formulas in this book. The authors and publisher are not responsible for any misuse or carelessness by the user or for allergic reactions.*

This book is dedicated to people who live in harmony with nature.
For only they are the truly free people on this earth.

CONTENTS

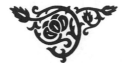

Acknowledgements

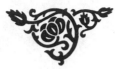

We would like to thank the following people for making this book possible:

* Ken Tamblyn for his valuable computer assistance.
* Paul Krohn and Jeffrey Schiller for all their help.
* All the librarians and staff at the Glendale Public Library in Glendale, Arizona.
* Special thanks to the people at Sterling Publishing Company, especially Sheila Anne Barry, acquisitions director, John Woodside, editorial director, and Jeanette Green, editor.
* Roslyn Blumenthal for her insight and guidance.

A Gift from Nature

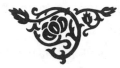

THE BRILLIANT colors of fragrant flowers, the energizing air from towering trees, and the house plants that purify our indoor air are just a few examples of nature's myriad benefits. But this is not all: plants do not only provide beauty and fresh air, they are necessary for our very existence. Without them, we would perish—lacking food to eat and oxygen to breathe.

Humans have always depended on a close relationship with nature. In order to survive, it was important to have an extensive knowledge of plant life in their immediate area to obtain food, medicine, clothing, and shelter. Humans have also discovered plant uses from close observation of animals. Sick sheep eat yarrow, lizards eat chamomile to relieve snakebites, cats and dogs chew grass to rid themselves of stomach problems, and bears eat bear's garlic as a spring tonic after awakening from hibernation. The instincts of animals to derive benefits from plants is one of the most fascinating aspects of nature.

Archaeological evidence found in Shanidar, Iraq, in 1975 indicates that Neanderthals used plants for food and medicine over 60,000 years ago. Discovered beside the ancient skeletal remains was pollen from eight species of medicinal plants, seven of which are still grown and used by Iraqi peasants today. The Ebers Papyrus, written by the Egyptians around 1550 BC, contains 877 prescriptions using medicinal plants.

Most populations in the Western world are concentrated in large cities today. Except for an occasional visit to a suburb or forest area, people live in an environment devoid of nature. While an urban life-style may be practical in economic terms, it can be disastrous for human health and well-being. As ailments caused by pollution and stress continue to rise annually, many people have turned to nature's herbs and essential oils to help reverse the harmful effects of urban life.

Essential oils are extracted from plants, shrubs, trees, flowers, seeds, roots, and grasses. These oils contain the essential life force of the plants. Aromatic oils promote plant growth, aid in reproduction by attracting pollinating insects, repel predators, and protect against disease. When we blend these wonderful, pure, and fragrant oils, they create the most enjoyable and effective products imaginable. The essences can be used for massage, skin and hair care, and as deodorants to keep fresh all day. When the oils are diffused or misted into the air, they produce an aroma that can smell like the perfume of a beautiful flower garden or the clean, fresh, invigorating air of a pine forest. You can also surrender yourself to the pleasures of relaxation and tranquility in a bath, foot bath, Jacuzzi, sauna, or steam room. In addition, you can treat yourself and your loved ones to a naturally fragrant home with scented candles, closets, drawers, laundry, carpets, and potpourri. Perhaps you would like to enjoy the outdoors without the fear of sunburning; carrier oils, such as jojoba, can help moisturize and protect your skin. Whatever formula you choose from this book, you will appreciate its use.

Those who use aromatic oils regularly hold them in high esteem. One can only respect the ability of essential oils to perform effectively, not just physically, but emotionally and spiritually. Even though these oils cannot completely substitute for interaction with nature, we can derive enormous benefits from their use. And they can relieve the unnatural experience of a city life that's divorced from trees, flowers, and plants.

Carol Schiller and David Schiller

500 Formulas for
AROMATHERAPY

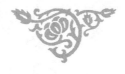

1

AROMATICS—PAST TO PRESENT

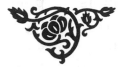

THE USE OF aromatic plants predates written records. Archaeological evidence indicates that the ancient civilizations of Egypt, Sumeria, Babylonia, Assyria, Crete, and China were skilled in extracting and blending plant oils and used ointments, fragrances, and incense. Aromatic plants were also used as medicinal remedies, and fragrant resins, gums, and woods were burned as incense during religious ceremonies as an offering for the gods.

Aromatics have been found in the tombs of Egyptian pharaohs, who lived more than 3,000 years ago. Ancient Egyptians soaked fragrant woods and resins in water and oil, then rubbed their bodies with the liquid. They also used these liquids to embalm the dead. Affluent women were so enthralled with the use of perfumes that they applied a different scent to each part of their bodies daily. Cleopatra, Egypt's famous queen, was a fragrance fanatic. She drenched the sails of her ship with perfumes to attract Mark Anthony.

The Greeks learned about the use of aromatics from the Egyptians. Greek athletes anointed themselves with fragrant oils to increase their strength for competitive games. After the Romans conquered Greece, they took full advantage of the many uses of aromatic oils as fragrances. They lavishly doused their bodies with perfume, scented their clothing, furniture, flags, military banners, and even the large amphitheatres. Roman soldiers were anointed with perfumes before battle. At one of Nero's feasts, a guest was asphyxiated by showers of rose fragrance. In the 1st century, Rome received between 2,500 and 3,000 tons of frankincense, and between 450 and 600 tons of myrrh from Arabia.

The fall of the Western Roman Empire brought an abrupt but temporary halt to the most extravagant use of aromatics ever seen. The city of Constantinople then became an important center of civilization, and its citizens in turn used aromatics lavishly. Overindulgence in fragrances by the general populace infuriated the Church, however. Perfume use became synonymous with degeneracy and immorality, and the early Church condemned the personal use of aromatics. Consequently, widespread use of plant oils ended in Europe. However, plant oil use continued in the Middle East and Far East.

In the 7th century, the Arabs continued the traditional art of perfumery and played an important role in introducing perfumes to other parts of the world. During the 10th century, Avicenna, an Arabian scientist, discovered the distillation process for extracting essences from plants and flowers. In the 13th century, the gallant knights and crusaders brought back scented gifts to Europe. As new trade routes to China and India opened, Europeans rekindled their passion for fragrances.

During the 14th century, the Black Death ravaged Europe and Asia, claiming millions of lives. The aromatic plants clove, cypress, cedar, pine, sage, rosemary, and thyme were burned in the streets, hospitals, and sickrooms in an attempt to ward off the infectious disease. Perfumers and those who were in daily contact with aromatic plants seemed immune to the plague.

The use of herbology and aromatics increased in popularity during the onset of yet another plague in Europe in 1665. It was recommended that every home burn aromatic substances to disinfect the air against the deadly bacteria. Aromatics reached another peak in 18th century France, during the reign of Louis XV. On festive occasions, even the water in Parisian fountains was perfumed. In his palace various perfumes were used daily.

In the mid-19th century, scientists began producing synthetic versions of essential plant oils, replacing these pure and precious natural oils that have been treasured for centuries.

Synthetic scents and fragrances are usually produced from petroleum derivatives and other synthetic materials. They not only pose harmful side effects for individuals using them, but processing these chemicals also pollutes the earth, water, and air. Essential oils, on the other hand, help balance the human body and work in harmony with nature. The use of these natural oils has gained popularity as more people become aware of their remarkable benefits. If we can use history as a guide to the future, perhaps people will rediscover what ancient people knew so well—the important value of plants and their valuable oils.

2

COMBINING SCENT AND TOUCH

THE SENSE OF SMELL

We think of the nose as primarily an organ of smell. However, its main function is moderating the temperature of inhaled air, which protects the linings of the lungs. Secondarily, the nose serves as a conduit that guides scent into the olfactory system. But only about 2 percent of inhaled air reaches the olfactory epithelium, which consists of two patches of tissue, covering an area of 1 square inch (2.5 square cm), in the upper rear of the nasal cavities. This is where we detect smell.

The olfactory nerve contains about 50 million smell receptors that protrude from mucous membranes. These hairs collect odors and convert them into messages which are relayed to the olfactory nerve and then to the brain for processing. Olfactory cells are the only nerve cells that are regenerated in the body.

Smell signals travel through the limbic system and play an important role in provoking feelings and memories. Among the structures that form the limbic system are the amygdala, where we process anger; the septum pellucidum, where we pro-

cess pleasurable sensations; and the hippocampus, which regulates how much attention we give these emotions and memories.

Since the sense of smell has a powerful impact on memory, odor can evoke the recall of emotions. The subconscious mind stores our memories of past experiences in a memory bank. When inhaling an aroma, the olfactory cells transmit a direct signal to the brain's memory bank. As this process occurs, a particular memory may be activated. If the scent is recognized, it may trigger a memory of past events and emotions associated with that particular odor. The smell memory may also trigger changes in body temperature, appetite, stress level, and sexual arousal. This close connection between smell and memory may help determine why certain individuals prefer one scent to another.

The chemical substances in scent that affect reproductive behavior and act as a sexual excitant are known as *pheromones*. Pheromones are present in perspiration, saliva, vaginal secretions, and urine. The apocrine glands, mainly located in the armpits and around the groin, produce pheromones. These glands are largest during a person's reproducing years. Secretions from the apocrine glands are odorless, however; odor occurs only after bacteria present react to the perspiration.

In one study, perspiration collected from men's underarms was swabbed three times a week on the upper lips of women whose menstrual cycles were less than 26 days or more than 33 days. After 3 months, all the women's cycles were regulated to 29.5 days—the optimum length for maximizing fertility. Menstrual cycles of women who live or work together become synchronized over a period of time. Many have speculated that this is due to a woman being exposed to another woman's perspiration (smelled over several months) and then adapting to the other woman's cycle. Men who are around women have more rapid hair growth, and women who are around men have more regulated cycles. Women are particularly sensitive to the odor of pheromones just before ovulation—about 1,000 times more so than at any other time during their cycle.

The most acute sense of smell known is that of the Chinese emperor moth, which can detect a scent it recognizes over 6 miles away. The male silkworm moth comes in a distant second, with its ability to detect the odor of the female silkworm's sexual secretion over 2 miles away. Although smell is not a highly developed human sense, smell remains nearly 10,000 times more sensitive than taste. Dogs are estimated to be over 1 million times more odor-sensitive than humans.

The connection between sex and scent in humans seems less important than it does for insects and animals. The pheromones that send an insect into a rage of passion do not affect humans the same way. Comparatively, humans do not demonstrate as intense or impulsive a response to scent signals from the opposite sex. Rats in the laboratory deprived of their sense of smell from birth, have low levels of growth hormones produced by the pituitary gland. Their growth is stunted and their testicles are subnormal. One out of 4 people who suffer from *anosmia* (loss or impairment of the sense of smell) lose interest in sexual activity. Hamsters that cannot smell their mates entirely lose interest in them.

Anosmia affects 2 million people in the United States. *Parosmia* is a common abnormality that causes a distorted sense of smell. The perception of a given scent may be interpreted as a consistent bad smell, similar to fecal matter. Both conditions, anosmia and parosmia, can result from head injuries or diseases.

Today, in our eagerness to deodorize our bodies and make them fragrant, we have disguised our natural odor communication. Nevertheless, we still communicate, but to a lesser extent, through our natural scents. To achieve a richer life, we must develop greater understanding of how scents affect our health and behavior. Only then will we begin to appreciate this most invaluable sense and become more conscious of its myriad messages.

THE SENSE OF TOUCH

Touch is a very important part of life. It is a language that communicates love, understanding, and reassurance and at the same time creates a comforting and healing effect. Many of us go through life being "touch starved" and rarely experience the wonderful feeling of being fully satisfied. Research in recent years has revealed that deprivation of touch can lead not only to emotional disturbance, but also to diminished intellectual ability, impaired physical growth, reduced sexual interest, and deterioration of the immune system. In addition, many forms of deviant behavior, such as those involving depression, violence, aggression, and hyperactivity have been traced to the lack of touch.

In a study conducted at the University of Wisconsin, baby monkeys deprived of their mother's bodily comfort grew up to be irritable, aggressive, and violent. When orphaned human babies have experienced deprivation of touch in orphanages, many wasted away and died of malnutrition. Newly born animals not licked by the mother shortly after birth usually die.

MASSAGE

For thousands of years, massage has been used as a therapeutic tool to nurture and heal the body. In Greece in the early 5th century BC, Hippocrates, the father of medicine, wrote about the benefits of massage. Asclepiades, an ancient Greek physician, challenged current medical thought after learning the value of massage and relied exclusively upon its use to restore and maintain health. The renowned Roman naturalist Pliny found relief from chronic asthma by having his body rubbed regularly. Julius Caesar was pinched daily all over his body to ease nerve pain and headaches from epilepsy.

During the Middle Ages, massage was almost forgotten until the French physician Ambroise Paré revived the art in the 16th century.

In the early 19th century, Per Henrik Ling, a Swedish fencing master and gymnastics instructor, used the massage technique *percussion* to overcome rheumatism. Recognizing the healing potential of massage, Ling combined its use with his teachings. Ling's efforts and dedication gained him official recognition, and in 1813 the Royal Gymnastic Central Institute, in Stockholm, sponsored by the Swedish government, included massage in its curriculum. After Ling's death in 1839, his former students published his work on massage. Massage gained popularity, thereafter, and institutes and spas opened in Germany, Austria, and France offering this therapy. This was the beginning of what is now known as Swedish massage.

In the United States, it wasn't until the early 1970s that people other than dancers, athletes, and members of spas and health clubs were aware of the benefits of massage. Massage is widely recognized today for its therapeutic value, and the practice continues to flourish in the Western World.

The Importance of Massage

The epidermis (outer layer of skin) and the layers beneath are designed to process sensation. Feeling is transmitted to the body and brain through an elaborate network of touch receptors to form natural electrical charges. The skin's sensitivity as well as its ability to relay tactile messages is why massage can improve gland, organ, and nerve function, while relaxing muscles and producing a positive emotional feeling. When touch, in the form of massage, is combined with essential oils, the results can be wonderful.

Preparing for a Massage

Be sure to avoid wounded areas and exercise special caution with pregnant women. To make massage more enjoyable, please follow these guidelines.

• The room for the massage should be comfortable, quiet, and warm, and provide a retreat from worldly stress and tensions.

• Continual concentration is necessary while giving a massage; therefore, chattering should be discouraged.

• Some people prefer to relax with soft music in the background.

• A soft, thick cushion draped with a towel or sheet may be used if a massage table is unavailable. If the massage is given on the floor, padding should extend beyond the person's body.

• Add a pleasant essential oil fragrance to the room before the treatment.

• Keep extra towels, blankets, and oil nearby to avoid searching for them during the treatment.

• Hands should be clean and warm before beginning the massage. Cold hands on a warm back are very uncomfortable and could make the body tense.

• Remove all jewelry.

• Wear comfortable, loose clothing.

• Warm the carrier oil (see massage oil section) that will be used by placing the container in warm water or near a heater. Pour a small amount into your palm, and rub both hands together until warmth is generated. Then massage the oil into the skin.

• It is important to feel relaxed while giving the massage, since tension can be transmitted to the person receiving the massage.

• If possible, maintain constant touch by gently resting one hand on the person receiving the massage when you move to a different position or side.

• Wash your hands at the end of the session.

Massage Therapies and Techniques

SWEDISH MASSAGE

Stroke Movements Slow, deliberate, continuous sequence, flowing.

Benefits Relaxing, relieves stress and tension, tones the muscles, improves circulation and lymph flow, and gives the mind and body an overall sense of well-being.

Oils Choose an aromatherapy massage formula listed in the Aromatherapy Formulas chapter. In order to grasp the muscles properly, the oil should be applied gradually throughout the treatment.

Massage Techniques

Step 1 **Gliding Stroke** Gently glide both hands over the skin, using long, broad, smooth strokes. Use this technique at the beginning and end of the treatment to relax the body. Whether you apply gentle or deep pressure depends on the person's preference and tolerance of pain.

Step 2 **Muscle Kneading** Use both hands alternately to grasp, lift, and gently squeeze the muscles in a continuous kneading motion, keeping your hands on the body at all times. The amount of pressure applied can be determined by the depth of penetration needed and the receiver's pain tolerance. Kneading movements should always be in the direction of the heart. This technique helps relax and tone the muscles.

Step 3 **Deep Tissue Pressure** Use the thumbs, fingertips, or heels of the hands to work deeper into the muscles and around the joints. With the fingertips or ball of each thumb, gradually press deeply into the muscle, using small, circular movements. It is important that you move the underlying tissue and do not slide your fingers across the skin. Avoid applying pressure on bony areas, such as the spine and rib cage.

Percussion This form of massage includes hacking, beating, and cupping. It may be used on soft tissue areas, such as the back (avoiding the spine), thighs, and buttocks. These strokes stimulate the body, break up congestion, and tone the muscles. As you begin a different stroke, maintain the same rhythm.

Hacking With the outside edge of both hands, alternately create a chopping motion directly on the muscles.

Beating With loosely clenched fists, alternately "beat" the muscles, using the fleshy side of the hand.

Cupping With your palms in a cupped position and the fingers held together, alternately "slap" the muscle area, which will create a loud sound.

Reflexology

Stroke Movements Slow.

Benefits Relaxing, relieves stress and tension, and revitalizes the body.

Oils Choose an aromatherapy massage formula, especially from the foot or hand rejuvenation category in the Aromatherapy Formulas chapter.

Powder For a dry massage, without oils, choose a foot powder from the formula section.

REFLEXOLOGY TECHNIQUES

Massage the entire hand or foot to encourage muscle relaxation. When the person becomes relaxed, apply direct and circular pressure alternately.

Direct Pressure Pinpoint a painful area using your thumb or fingertip. Gently apply pressure directly on the sensitive point and hold your thumb or finger down firmly for several seconds. Release, then reapply pressure again. As you repeat this technique, gradually increase the amount of pressure according to the person's pain tolerance.

Circular Pressure Slowly rotate your thumb or fingertip in a circular motion over the entire foot. As you find painful areas, press down firmly into the spot and manipulate the reflex point with circular movements. Gradually increase the amount of pressure according to the person's pain tolerance.

CAUTION Do not use reflexology on a pregnant woman. Certain reflex points can trigger the onset of childbirth.

3

SELECTING AND USING PURE OILS

SAFETY GUIDELINES AND HELPFUL HINTS

Essential oils can be extremely beneficial when used properly. Be sure to follow these guidelines.

• Since essential oils are highly concentrated substances, always dilute them in a *carrier oil*, such as sweet almond, grapeseed, flaxseed, or sesame, before using them on the skin. Add extra carrier oil to a blend that's applied near sensitive areas, like the eyes, lips, or genitals. If any skin irritation occurs when using essential oils, quickly soothe the area by immediately applying lavender oil, "neat," or a carrier oil such as jojoba.

• Carrier oils protect and help soothe the skin tissue and can be applied directly anywhere on the body.

• When using essential oils, be careful not to get the oils or their strong vapors in your eyes. If this happens, flush the eyes with cool water or apply a drop of sweet almond oil.

• Do not consume alcohol (other than a glass of wine with a meal) when using essential oils.

• Pregnant women should take extra care when using essential oils. These oils are considered safe when used in small amounts:

Cardamom, coriander, geranium, ginger, grapefruit, lavender, lemon, lemongrass, lime, mandarin, melissa, neroli, palmarosa, petitgrain, spearmint, ylang-ylang

• For someone who tends to be highly allergic, here's a simple test to determine if he or she is sensitive to a particular oil. First, rub a drop of carrier oil into the upper chest. In 12 hours, check for redness or other skin irritation. If the skin remains clear, place 1 drop of selected essential oil in 15 drops of the same carrier oil, and again rub it into the upper chest. If no skin reaction appears after 12 hours, it's probably safe to use both the carrier oil and the essential oil.

• After applying citrus oils to the skin,

avoid exposure to sunlight, since the oil may burn the skin.

• Since these oils tend to be irritating to the skin, take extra care when using them, especially if you have dry skin:

Cinnamon, clove, grapefruit, lemon, lemongrass, lime, mandarin, melissa, orange, black pepper, peppermint, spearmint

• If a person has sensitive skin, the essential oils in the bath, foot and hand baths, and massage oil formulas should be reduced to half strength.

• The essential oils should not be used while a person is on medication—in order for the oils not to interfere with the medicine.

• Store essential oils out of reach and out of sight of children.

• Light and oxygen cause oils to deteriorate rapidly, so always store them in brown glass bottles, in a cool, dark place. Although refrigeration does not prevent spoilage, it diminishes the speed at which the spoilage occurs.

• Keep bottles tightly closed to prevent the volatile oils from evaporating and oxidizing.

• When spilled on furniture, many essential oils will remove the finish. It's best to be careful when handling the bottles.

• The shelf life for refined carrier oils is about a year. Since unrefined oils have a shorter shelf life, store in the freezer and refrigerate after opening.

The shelf life for most essential oils is about 1 to 2 years. However, citrus oils only stay fresh 6 to 9 months.

• The resins of benzoin, Peru balsam, and tolu balsam can be thick and sticky and, therefore, difficult to use. To make them more workable, place a small piece of beeswax into an empty glass baby food jar. Put the jar into a pan of water and heat on a low flame. When the wax liquifies, add the resin and an equal amount of carrier oil and stir well. Remove the jar from the heated pan and allow to cool for several minutes before adding the essential oils.

EXTRACTION PROCESSES

The extraction process helps determine the purity of the oil. It is advisable to become knowledgeable about the various methods of extraction before purchasing carrier and essential oils.

Steam Distillation   In this method, steam from boiling water is used to extract the essential oils from the plant material. Then, the steam is cooled and condensed into a liquid from which the oil is skimmed off as it floats on top of the water. Aromatherapists prefer steam distillation since it produces a good quality of essential oil.

Expeller, Mechanically, or Cold Pressed Seeds, nuts, fruits, and vegetables are pressed without the use of heat; however, a large percentage of these oils are usually refined afterwards using high heat and harsh chemicals. (See Refining Process of Carrier Oils).

Maceration   Flowers are soaked in hot oil until the cells rupture and the oil absorbs the essence.

Solvent Extraction Solvents, such as hexane and other toxic chemicals, are used to extract the oil from the plant material. This method is less costly than other methods, and efficiently produces a greater amount of oil. However, toxic residues *remain* in the oil, which makes the resulting product undesirable for those who seek pure oils. Absolute flower oils and nearly all vegetable oils are extracted by this method.

Refining Process of Carrier Oils After the oil has been extracted from the plant material, it is usually refined. The refining process includes these steps:

Degumming This process removes chlorophyll, lecithin, vitamins, and minerals from the oil.

Refining An alkaline solution, sodium hydroxide (lye), is added to refine the oil.

Bleaching Fuller's Earth is added as a bleaching agent and then filtered out, further removing nutritive substances. The oil at this stage turns clear.

Deodorizing The oil is deodorized by steam distillation at high temperatures over 450 degrees F (230 degrees C) for 30 to 60 minutes.

Winterizing The oil is cooled and again filtered. This process prevents the oil from becoming cloudy during cold temperatures. The finished product is nutrient-deficient; only fatty acids remain.

Several synthetic antioxidants are usually added to replace the natural antioxidants present in the oil prior to the refining process.

SELECTING QUALITY OILS

Never use synthetic oils and oils extracted by chemical solvents. Many synthetic oils on the market today replicate the fragrances of natural oils, and many people unknowingly use them, hoping to derive their benefits. The synthetic chemicals that create these products do not contain the beneficial properties of pure plant oils. In addition, many synthetic compounds can be very irritating to the body and nervous system. Oils extracted with solvents contain toxic residues harmful to the body. It is important to select *unrefined* carrier oils, and essential oils extracted by *steam distillation* or which have been *pressed mechanically* or by an *expeller.*

SUBSTITUTIONS FOR OILS

Many essential oils in this book are quite expensive. In order to economize in making the blends, you can substitute oils and still derive up to 90 percent of the benefits of the original formulas.

Original Oil	Substitute Oil(s)
Jasmine	Ylang-ylang
Neroli	Mandarin + Petitgrain (equal parts)
Chamomile	Lavender
Rose	Bois de rose
Bergamot	Grapefruit
Tea tree	Cajeput + Lavender (equal parts)

Melissa	Lemon + Petitgrain (equal parts)
Sandalwood	Benzoin + Cedar-wood (equal parts)
Clary sage	Sage + Nutmeg (equal parts)
Myrrh	Myrrh oil blend

Myrrh Oil Blend Here's an inexpensive way to make your own myrrh oil blend. Purchase myrrh resin or powder and finely grind it in a coffee mill. Then add the fine powder to a carrier oil. Heat the mixture for 30 minutes and allow to sit for a few days before using. If the blend feels gritty, filter the oil through a coffee filter.

Other Substitutions

You may also substitute these essential oils for each other (lemon for lime or lime for lemon):

Lemon——Lime
Spearmint——Peppermint
Orange——Mandarin
Grapefruit——Lemon

DROP EQUIVALENTS

20 drops	= 1/5 teaspoon	= 1 ml
100 drops	= 1 teaspoon	= 5 ml
300 drops	= 1 tablespoon	= 15 ml
600 drops	= 1 ounce	= 30 ml

4

AROMATHERAPY FORMULAS

Please review safety guidelines and helpful hints in the Selecting and Using Pure Oils chapter before using the essential oils. Also be sure to follow the blending directions listed in each section for proper use of the formulas.

AIR FRESHENERS

Many of us have experienced elevated moods from smelling the beautiful fragrances of flowers, feeling an ocean breeze, and breathing fresh forest air. Living in big cities, we are deprived of these natural aromas every day. With the use of essential oils, we can recreate the scents we enjoy and bring nature into our homes and offices to enhance our lives.

For All Air Fresheners   Fill a 4-fluid ounce (120 ml) mist spray bottle with purified water, and add the essential oils. Tighten the cap, shake well, and spray the mist into the air. As the mist ages inside the bottle, the scent improves and becomes stronger.

✦ Citrus ✦

lime	50 drops	orange	50 drops
grapefruit	50 drops	lemon	35 drops
orange	10 drops	grapefruit	20 drops
patchouli	10 drops	cedarwood	15 drops
pure water	4 fluid ounces (120 ml)	pure water	4 fluid ounces (120 ml)

✦ ✦ ✦   ✦ ✦ ✦

✦ Citrus (continued) ✦

bergamot	50 drops	lime	40 drops
mandarin	50 drops	lemon	40 drops
clove	20 drops	petitgrain	20 drops
pure water	4 fluid ounces (120 ml)	benzoin	20 drops
		pure water	4 fluid ounces (120 ml)

✦ Floral ✦

orange	50 drops	geranium	35 drops
rose	25 drops	bois de rose	25 drops
clove	20 drops	rose	25 drops
cinnamon	15 drops	clove	20 drops
jasmine	10 drops	Peru balsam	15 drops
pure water	4 fluid ounces (120 ml)	pure water	4 fluid ounces (120 ml)

✦ ✦ ✦

rose	75 drops	ylang-ylang	50 drops
orange	25 drops	geranium	25 drops
clove	20 drops	petitgrain	25 drops
pure water	4 fluid ounces (120 ml)	tolu balsam	20 drops
		pure water	4 fluid ounces (120 ml)

✦ Forest ✦

spruce .... 50 drops

lavender .... 25 drops

eucalyptus .... 25 drops

cedarwood .... 20 drops

pure water .... 4 fluid ounces (120 ml)

✦ ✦ ✦

pine .... 40 drops

cajeput .... 40 drops

cypress .... 20 drops

sandalwood .... 20 drops

pure water .... 4 fluid ounces (120 ml)

rosemary .... 30 drops

spruce .... 30 drops

myrtle .... 30 drops

lime .... 15 drops

patchouli .... 15 drops

pure water .... 4 fluid ounces (120 ml)

✦ ✦ ✦

spruce .... 40 drops

bois de rose .... 30 drops

spearmint .... 30 drops

eucalyptus .... 20 drops

pure water .... 4 fluid ounces (120 ml)

✦ Mint ✦

peppermint .... 40 drops

caraway .... 40 drops

petitgrain .... 20 drops

spearmint .... 10 drops

patchouli .... 10 drops

pure water .... 4 fluid ounces (120 ml)

✦ ✦ ✦

peppermint .... 50 drops

spearmint .... 50 drops

Peru balsam .... 20 drops

pure water .... 4 fluid ounces (120 ml)

spearmint .... 40 drops

lavender .... 30 drops

rosemary .... 20 drops

benzoin .... 10 drops

peppermint .... 10 drops

lime .... 10 drops

pure water .... 4 fluid ounces (120 ml)

✦ ✦ ✦

peppermint .... 75 drops

eucalyptus .... 35 drops

clove .... 10 drops

pure water .... 4 fluid ounces (120 ml)

✦ Spice ✦

caraway .... 35 drops

anise .... 20 drops

cinnamon .... 20 drops

ginger .... 20 drops

clove .... 15 drops

lime .... 10 drops

pure water .... 4 fluid ounces (120 ml)

✦ ✦ ✦

peppermint .... 30 drops

thyme .... 30 drops

cumin .... 30 drops

patchouli .... 20 drops

allspice .... 10 drops

pure water .... 4 fluid ounces (120 ml)

rosemary .... 30 drops

coriander .... 25 drops

allspice .... 25 drops

cumin .... 20 drops

clove .... 20 drops

pure water .... 4 fluid ounces (120 ml)

✦ ✦ ✦

marjoram .... 25 drops

sage .... 25 drops

spearmint .... 25 drops

clove .... 25 drops

patchouli .... 20 drops

pure water .... 4 fluid ounces (120 ml)

Aroma Lamps

An aroma lamp can be ceramic, marble, glass, or porcelain. It has a small container that is filled with water and is heated by a candle. When essential oils are added to water, aromatic vapor is dispersed into the air. About 15 to 20 drops of essential oil can be used at one time.

Inhale the vapors deeply for best results.

✦ Breathe More Easily ✦

myrtle	5 drops	pine	6 drops
lemongrass	5 drops	lavender	5 drops
allspice	5 drops	eucalyptus	4 drops
cajeput	5 drops	cubeb	4 drops
		lime	1 drop

✦ ✦ ✦

clove	4 drops		
cajeput	4 drops	lemon	5 drops
myrtle	4 drops	pine	5 drops
spruce	4 drops	lavender	5 drops
lemon	4 drops	spearmint	5 drops

✦ ✦ ✦

spearmint	6 drops	rosemary	5 drops
marjoram	4 drops	cubeb	5 drops
rosemary	4 drops	pine	5 drops
cubeb	4 drops	grapefruit	5 drops
lime	2 drops		

✦ Room Disinfectant ✦

pine	6 drops	lemon	5 drops
cinnamon	6 drops	tea tree	5 drops
juniper berries	5 drops	sage	5 drops
clove	3 drops	cajeput	5 drops

✦ ✦ ✦　　　　　　✦ ✦ ✦

✦ Room Disinfectant (continued) ✦

eucalyptus	6 drops		clove	6 drops
thyme	6 drops		lime	5 drops
clove	3 drops		allspice	4 drops
lemon	3 drops		cinnamon	4 drops
cinnamon	2 drops		lemon	1 drop

✦ Refreshing ✦

lime	8 drops		pine	8 drops
spearmint	8 drops		spearmint	8 drops
myrtle	4 drops		palmarosa	4 drops

✦ ✦ ✦

peppermint	8 drops		grapefruit	8 drops
eucalyptus	8 drops		bergamot	4 drops
lemongrass	4 drops		ginger	4 drops
			clove	4 drops

✦ Romance ✦

caraway	5 drops		clary sage	5 drops
patchouli	5 drops		clove	5 drops
orange	5 drops		ylang-ylang	5 drops
benzoin	5 drops		black pepper	5 drops

✦ ✦ ✦

sandalwood	7 drops		ylang-ylang	7 drops
ylang-ylang	7 drops		palmarosa	7 drops
orange	6 drops		bergamot	6 drops

Aroma Lamps

✦ Stress Reduction ✦

melissa	10 drops		lavender	10 drops
allspice	10 drops		mandarin	10 drops

✦   ✦   ✦

sandalwood	10 drops		chamomile	9 drops
lavender	5 drops		cinnamon	6 drops
spruce	5 drops		fennel	5 drops

✦ Baby Oil ✦

To help protect and soothe your baby's skin from diaper rash, use one of these lavender blends. Apply an ample amount of baby oil on the baby's skin, and store the remaining oil for the next application.

lavender .... 5 drops		*lavender* .... 5 drops
hazelnut .... 2 tablespoons (30 ml)		*olive* .... 2 tablespoons (30 ml)
✦ ✦ ✦		✦ ✦ ✦
lavender .... 5 drops		*lavender* .... 5 drops
flaxseed .... 2 tablespoons (30 ml)		*sesame* .... 2 tablespoons (30 ml)

✦ Baby Powder ✦

bois de rose .... 5 drops	*lavender* .... 5 drops
cornstarch .... 2 tablespoons (30 ml)	*cornstarch* .... 2 tablespoons (30 ml)

BATHS

Besides being necessary for proper hygiene, baths are beneficial to improve one's health. When aromatic oils are added to the bath water, they can help you feel move relaxed and stress-free.

As you prepare your bath, close the window and door to prevent the oil vapors from escaping. Fill the bathtub with warm/hot water. To soften your skin and remove impurities, dissolve 1 cup of epsom salt in the bath water. Then dilute the essential oils in any of these carrier oils: grapeseed, sweet almond, hazelnut, or sesame. Pour the blend into the water. Swirl the water to disperse the oil evenly. Enter the bath immediately, since essential oils evaporate quickly. Relax and enjoy the bath for at least 30 minutes.

✦ Breathe More Easily ✦

cajeput .... 5 drops	*spruce* .... 5 drops
eucalyptus .... 5 drops	*lavender* .... 5 drops
peppermint .... 5 drops	*cajeput* .... 5 drops
carrier oil .... 1 teaspoon (5 ml)	*carrier oil* .... 1 teaspoon (5 ml)

✦ ✦ ✦

myrtle .... 4 drops	*eucalyptus* .... 4 drops
spruce .... 4 drops	*chamomile* .... 4 drops
rosemary .... 4 drops	*anise* .... 3 drops
grapefruit .... 3 drops	*lemon* .... 3 drops
carrier oil .... 1 teaspoon (5 ml)	*petitgrain* .... 1 drop
	carrier oil .... 1 teaspoon (5 ml)

✦ ✦ ✦ (left) / ✦ ✦ ✦ (right)

myrtle .... 5 drops	*lavender* .... 5 drops
lavender .... 5 drops	*cajeput* .... 5 drops
marjoram .... 3 drops	*grapefruit* .... 5 drops
benzoin .... 2 drops	*carrier oil* .... 1 teaspoon (5 ml)
carrier oil .... 1 teaspoon (5 ml)	

✦ Calming ✦

petitgrain .... 5 drops

lavender .... 5 drops

fennel .... 3 drops

orange .... 2 drops

carrier oil .... 1 teaspoon (5 ml)

✦ ✦ ✦

cypress .... 5 drops

marjoram .... 3 drops

melissa .... 3 drops

lemon .... 3 drops

geranium .... 1 drop

carrier oil .... 1 teaspoon (5 ml)

✦ ✦ ✦

allspice .... 5 drops

chamomile .... 5 drops

mandarin .... 5 drops

carrier oil .... 1 teaspoon (5 ml)

petitgrain .... 5 drops

ylang-ylang .... 5 drops

orange .... 5 drops

carrier oil .... 1 teaspoon (5 ml)

✦ ✦ ✦

geranium .... 5 drops

sandalwood .... 5 drops

lemon .... 5 drops

carrier oil .... 1 teaspoon (5 ml)

✦ ✦ ✦

chamomile .... 5 drops

geranium .... 5 drops

clary sage .... 2 drops

lemon .... 2 drops

Peru balsam .... 1 drop

carrier oil .... 1 teaspoon (5 ml)

✦ Mood Elevating ✦

bois de rose .... 5 drops

palmarosa .... 5 drops

grapefruit .... 3 drops

petitgrain .... 2 drops

carrier oil .... 1 teaspoon (5 ml)

✦ ✦ ✦

geranium .... 5 drops

bergamot .... 4 drops

allspice .... 3 drops

orange .... 3 drops

carrier oil .... 1 teaspoon (5 ml)

✦ ✦ ✦

BATHS

ylang-ylang .... 5 drops	bergamot .... 5 drops
sandalwood .... 5 drops	rosemary .... 5 drops
grapefruit .... 5 drops	benzoin .... 5 drops
carrier oil .... 1 teaspoon (5 ml)	carrier oil .... 1 teaspoon (5 ml)

✦ ✦ ✦

clary sage .... 3 drops	patchouli .... 4 drops
bois de rose .... 3 drops	bergamot .... 3 drops
lime .... 3 drops	clary sage .... 3 drops
patchouli .... 3 drops	geranium .... 3 drops
geranium .... 3 drops	palmarosa .... 2 drops
carrier oil .... 1 teaspoon (5 ml)	carrier oil .... 1 teaspoon (5 ml)

✦ Muscle Relaxers ✦

cedarwood .... 4 drops	cypress .... 5 drops
chamomile .... 4 drops	marjoram .... 3 drops
lavender .... 4 drops	lavender .... 3 drops
lemongrass .... 3 drops	sweet basil .... 2 drops
carrier oil .... 1 teaspoon (5 ml)	cedarwood .... 2 drops
	carrier oil .... 1 teaspoon (5 ml)

✦ ✦ ✦

cypress .... 5 drops	
sandalwood .... 5 drops	allspice .... 5 drops
nutmeg .... 3 drops	petitgrain .... 5 drops
lavender .... 2 drops	ylang-ylang .... 5 drops
carrier oil .... 1 teaspoon (5 ml)	carrier oil .... 1 teaspoon (5 ml)

✦ Premenstrual Syndrome ✦

bergamot .... 5 drops
geranium .... 5 drops
palmarosa .... 5 drops
carrier oil .... 1 teaspoon (5 ml)

✦　✦　✦

bergamot .... 4 drops
fennel .... 4 drops
bois de rose .... 4 drops
melissa .... 3 drops
carrier oil .... 1 teaspoon (5 ml)

grapefruit .... 4 drops
clary sage .... 4 drops
ylang-ylang .... 4 drops
geranium .... 3 drops
carrier oil .... 1 teaspoon (5 ml)

✦　✦　✦

allspice .... 5 drops
lemon .... 4 drops
chamomile .... 3 drops
geranium .... 3 drops
carrier oil .... 1 teaspoon (5 ml)

✦ Refreshing ✦

bergamot .... 4 drops
eucalyptus .... 4 drops
melissa .... 4 drops
peppermint .... 3 drops
carrier oil .... 1 teaspoon (5 ml)

✦　✦　✦

lavender .... 5 drops
bergamot .... 3 drops
lime .... 3 drops
cypress .... 2 drops
cajeput .... 2 drops
carrier oil .... 1 teaspoon (5 ml)

lavender .... 5 drops
peppermint .... 4 drops
grapefruit .... 3 drops
lemongrass .... 3 drops
carrier oil .... 1 teaspoon (5 ml)

✦　✦　✦

spruce .... 4 drops
geranium .... 4 drops
spearmint .... 4 drops
juniper berries .... 2 drops
lemon .... 2 drops
carrier oil .... 1 teaspoon (5 ml)

BATHS

✦ Stress Relievers ✦

allspice	5 drops		sandalwood	5 drops
rosemary	4 drops		fennel	3 drops
fennel	2 drops		melissa	3 drops
cypress	2 drops		sweet basil	2 drops
mandarin	2 drops		lavender	2 drops
carrier oil	1 teaspoon (5ml)		carrier oil	1 teaspoon (5ml)

✦ ✦ ✦   ✦ ✦ ✦

lavender	3 drops		marjoram	4 drops
chamomile	3 drops		cedarwood	4 drops
melissa	3 drops		melissa	3 drops
cedarwood	3 drops		grapefruit	2 drops
mandarin	3 drops		orange	2 drops
carrier oil	1 teaspoon (5ml)		carrier oil	1 teaspoon (5ml)

Body Powder

Measure the amount of cornstarch and pour into a widemouthed glass jar or a spice powder container; then add the essential oils. Tighten the cap and let the body powder sit for a day. Shake well before using.

✦ Citrus Scent ✦

mandarin .... 12 drops	bergamot .... 15 drops
lemon .... 12 drops	grapefruit .... 10 drops
patchouli .... 6 drops	sandalwood .... 5 drops
cornstarch .... 2 tablespoons (30 ml)	cornstarch .... 2 tablespoons (30 ml)

✦ ✦ ✦

petitgrain .... 15 drops	grapefruit .... 15 drops
neroli .... 15 drops	lime .... 10 drops
cornstarch .... 2 tablespoons (30 ml)	allspice .... 5 drops
	cornstarch .... 2 tablespoons (30 ml)

✦ ✦ ✦

lime .... 10 drops	
orange .... 10 drops	lemon .... 20 drops
clove .... 5 drops	lavender .... 5 drops
petitgrain .... 5 drops	allspice .... 5 drops
cornstarch .... 2 tablespoons (30 ml)	cornstarch .... 2 tablespoons (30 ml)

✦ Floral Scent ✦

bois de rose .... 10 drops	ylang-ylang .... 10 drops
lavender .... 10 drops	melissa .... 5 drops
mandarin .... 5 drops	clove .... 5 drops
ylang-ylang .... 5 drops	nutmeg .... 5 drops
cornstarch .... 2 tablespoons (30 ml)	orange .... 5 drops
	cornstarch .... 2 tablespoons (30 ml)

✦ ✦ ✦

✦ ✦ ✦

BODY POWDER

jasmine .... 10 drops

bois de rose .... 10 drops

rose .... 5 drops

clove .... 5 drops

cornstarch .... 2 tablespoons (30 ml)

✦ ✦ ✦

rose .... 20 drops

orange .... 10 drops

cornstarch .... 2 tablespoons (30 ml)

geranium .... 10 drops

bergamot .... 10 drops

ylang-ylang .... 10 drops

cornstarch .... 2 tablespoons (30 ml)

✦ ✦ ✦

ylang-ylang .... 20 drops

geranium .... 10 drops

cornstarch .... 2 tablespoons (30 ml)

✦ Forest Scent ✦

spruce .... 10 drops

cedarwood .... 10 drops

juniper berries .... 5 drops

cajeput .... 5 drops

cornstarch .... 2 tablespoons (30 ml)

✦ ✦ ✦

pine .... 15 drops

spruce .... 10 drops

spearmint .... 5 drops

cornstarch .... 2 tablespoons (30 ml)

✦ ✦ ✦

eucalyptus .... 10 drops

juniper berries .... 10 drops

myrtle .... 5 drops

lemon .... 5 drops

cornstarch .... 2 tablespoons (30 ml)

sandalwood .... 10 drops

chamomile .... 10 drops

rosemary .... 5 drops

lemon .... 5 drops

cornstarch .... 2 tablespoons (30 ml)

✦ ✦ ✦

cypress .... 10 drops

eucalyptus .... 10 drops

sandalwood .... 10 drops

cornstarch .... 2 tablespoons (30 ml)

✦ ✦ ✦

sage .... 10 drops

patchouli .... 5 drops

cedarwood .... 5 drops

spruce .... 5 drops

lavender .... 5 drops

cornstarch .... 2 tablespoons (30 ml)

BODY POWDER

✦ Minty Scent ✦

peppermint	10 drops		spearmint	15 drops
spruce	10 drops		lemon	5 drops
clove	5 drops		patchouli	5 drops
spearmint	5 drops		lavender	5 drops
cornstarch	2 tablespoons (30 ml)		cornstarch	2 tablespoons (30 ml)

✦ ✦ ✦

peppermint	15 drops		spearmint	15 drops
caraway	10 drops		lavender	10 drops
lavender	5 drops		sweet bay	5 drops
cornstarch	2 tablespoons (30 ml)		cornstarch	2 tablespoons (30 ml)

✦ Spicy Scent ✦

allspice	15 drops		caraway	10 drops
caraway	10 drops		clove	10 drops
lavender	5 drops		rosemary	10 drops
cornstarch	2 tablespoons (30 ml)		cornstarch	2 tablespoons (30 ml)

BREATH FRESHENERS

Mix all ingredients in a mist sprayer, shake well before using, then mist once or twice directly into the mouth.

peppermint .... 10 drops

spearmint .... 10 drops

pure water .... 4 fluid ounces (120 ml)

honey .... 1/2 teaspoon (2.5 ml)

✦ ✦ ✦

peppermint .... 10 drops

lavender .... 5 drops

clove .... 5 drops

pure water .... 4 fluid ounces (120 ml)

honey .... 1/2 teaspoon (2.5 ml)

✦ ✦ ✦

pine .... 10 drops

anise .... 5 drops

lavender .... 5 drops

pure water .... 4 fluid ounces (120 ml)

honey .... 1/2 teaspoon (2.5 ml)

✦ ✦ ✦

lemon .... 10 drops

lavender .... 10 drops

pure water .... 4 fluid ounces (120 ml)

honey .... 1/2 teaspoon (2.5 ml)

cinnamon .... 10 drops

orange .... 10 drops

pure water .... 4 fluid ounces (120 ml)

honey .... 1/2 teaspoon (2.5 ml)

✦ ✦ ✦

spearmint .... 10 drops

lime .... 10 drops

pure water .... 4 fluid ounces (120 ml)

honey .... 1/2 teaspoon (2.5 ml)

✦ ✦ ✦

allspice .... 10 drops

lemon .... 5 drops

anise .... 5 drops

pure water .... 4 fluid ounces (120 ml)

honey .... 1/2 teaspoon (2.5 ml)

✦ ✦ ✦

chamomile .... 10 drops

allspice .... 5 drops

pine .... 5 drops

pure water .... 4 fluid ounces (120 ml)

honey .... 1/2 teaspoon (2.5 ml)

Candles

You can create a delightful atmosphere by burning a candle scented with essential oils.

Place several drops of the oil on the wax before lighting the candle. Avoid dropping the oil into the flame or on the wick. For thick candles, heat a metal ice pick and pierce a hole through the wax and add essential oils. Select your favorite oil(s) from one of the scent categories.

Citrus Scent	Floral Scent	Forest Scent	Minty Scent	Spicy Scent
grapefruit	benzoin	eucalyptus	peppermint	allspice
lemon	jasmine	myrtle	spearmint	caraway
lemongrass	rose	pine		clove
lime	tolu balsam	rosemary		sage
melissa	ylang-ylang	spruce		
neroli				
orange				

CARPET FRESHENERS

Mix all ingredients in a widemouthed glass jar and tighten the cap. Set aside for 24 hours to allow the aromas to permeate the powder. Sprinkle over carpeting, leave for 10 to 15 minutes, and vacuum.

lavender	60 drops
cinnamon	20 drops
orange	20 drops
bicarbonate of soda	1/2 cup (120 ml)

◆ ◆ ◆

clove	60 drops
peppermint	20 drops
dill	20 drops
bicarbonate of soda	1/2 cup (120 ml)

◆ ◆ ◆

lime	50 drops
orange	30 drops
patchouli	20 drops
bicarbonate of soda	1/2 cup (120 ml)

rosemary	60 drops
spruce	30 drops
orange	10 drops
bicarbonate of soda	1/2 cup (120 ml)

◆ ◆ ◆

eucalyptus	30 drops
cinnamon	30 drops
lemongrass	30 drops
clove	10 drops
bicarbonate of soda	1/2 cup (120 ml)

◆ ◆ ◆

anise	40 drops
clove	40 drops
patchouli	20 drops
bicarbonate of soda	1/2 cup (120 ml)

CHAPPED LIPS

Apply aloe vera gel to your chapped lips before using one of these moisturizing formulas.

lavender .... 3 drops	*lavender* .... 3 drops
sandalwood .... 2 drops	*bois de rose* .... 2 drops
macadamia .... 1 teaspoon (5 ml)	*flaxseed* .... 1 teaspoon (5 ml)

✦ ✦ ✦

chamomile .... 3 drops	*neroli* .... 3 drops
benzoin .... 2 drops	*Peru balsam* .... 2 drops
sesame .... 1 teaspoon (5 ml)	*sweet almond* .... 1 teaspoon (5 ml)

✦ ✦ ✦

bois de rose .... 3 drops	*chamomile* .... 3 drops
geranium .... 2 drops	*sandalwood* .... 2 drops
sweet almond .... 1 teaspoon (5 ml)	*flaxseed* .... 1 teaspoon (5 ml)

CLOSET AND DRAWER SCENTS

Put 10 drops of your favorite essential oil on a cotton ball and place it inside a plastic bag. Leave the bag open and place it in a closet or dresser drawer to scent your clothing. When the scent wears off, repeat again with additional drops.

DEODORANTS

✦ Foot Deodorizer ✦

Some people experience unpleasant odors from their feet. These formulas will keep the feet smelling fresh. Select one of the formulas, and use the entire blend on each foot. Finish by dabbing on cornstarch to dry any remaining oil on the skin. Apply daily if needed.

flaxseed	20 drops	*flaxseed*	20 drops
tolu balsam	3 drops	*tolu balsam*	3 drops
cypress	2 drops	*bergamot*	3 drops
lavender	2 drops		

✦ Underarm Deodorants ✦

One application of one of these natural deodorants will keep you smelling nice for up to 2 days. First apply jojoba oil. Select a formula and use the entire blend on each underarm. Rub in well and wipe off any excess oil with a tissue. Finish by dabbing on cornstarch to dry any remaining oil. Make sure to remove any excess residue to avoid staining your clothing. After a woman shaves her underarms, she should wait at least 30 minutes before applying the deodorant.

tolu balsam	3 drops	*tolu balsam*	3 drops
lavender	2 drops	*petitgrain*	2 drops

Diffusers

Diffusers have become popular during the last few years. These devices disperse a fine mist of the microparticles of essential oils, which purifies and revitalizes the indoor atmosphere. Electric diffusers are especially wonderful for large rooms and office buildings, since the mist is continuously diffused into the air.

Thick or resinous oils will cause damage to the nebulizer; therefore, choose from the following oils.

Breathe More Easily	Disinfectant	Energizing	Stress-Free
cajeput	*allspice*	*eucalyptus*	*allspice*
clove	*bergamot*	*lemon*	*bois de rose*
eucalyptus	*cajeput*	*lime*	*chamomile*
juniper berries	*cinnamon*	*peppermint*	*geranium*
lavender	*clove*	*pine*	*grapefruit*
myrtle	*eucalyptus*	*spearmint*	*lavender*
peppermint	*lavender*		*lemon*
pine	*pine*		*mandarin*
spearmint	*rosemary*		*melissa*
spruce	*sage*		*neroli*
tea tree	*tea tree*		*orange*
	thyme		*petitgrain*

FOOT BATHS

Select a carrier oil—grapeseed, sweet almond, hazelnut, or sesame—to dilute the essential oils. Then fill the basin with warm water, and add one of the formulas below. Swirl the water to disperse the blended oils and relax for at least 15 minutes.

✦ Rejuvenating ✦

lemon	5 drops
spearmint	4 drops
black pepper	3 drops
pine	3 drops
carrier oil	1 teaspoon (5 ml)

✦ ✦ ✦

cubeb	3 drops
geranium	3 drops
thyme	3 drops
allspice	3 drops
pine	3 drops
carrier oil	1 teaspoon (5 ml)

✦ ✦ ✦

cypress	4 drops
lemon	4 drops
palmarosa	3 drops
cinnamon	2 drops
eucalyptus	2 drops
carrier oil	1 teaspoon (5 ml)

✦ ✦ ✦

eucalyptus	4 drops
pine	4 drops
peppermint	4 drops
geranium	3 drops
carrier oil	1 teaspoon (5 ml)

ginger	4 drops
lime	4 drops
geranium	4 drops
spearmint	3 drops
carrier oil	1 teaspoon (5 ml)

✦ ✦ ✦

myrtle	4 drops
spearmint	4 drops
grapefruit	4 drops
cajeput	3 drops
carrier oil	1 teaspoon (5 ml)

✦ ✦ ✦

sandalwood	3 drops
black pepper	3 drops
spruce	3 drops
geranium	3 drops
grapefruit	3 drops
carrier oil	1 teaspoon (5 ml)

✦ ✦ ✦

thyme	3 drops
peppermint	3 drops
lemongrass	3 drops
geranium	3 drops
lavender	3 drops
carrier oil	1 teaspoon (5 ml)

✦ Relaxing ✦

mandarin .... 4 drops
lavender .... 4 drops
anise .... 2 drops
sweet basil .... 2 drops
petitgrain .... 2 drops
lemon .... 1 drop
carrier oil .... 1 teaspoon (5 ml)

✦　✦　✦

frankincense .... 4 drops
neroli .... 4 drops
anise .... 4 drops
lemon .... 3 drops
carrier oil .... 1 teaspoon (5 ml)

✦　✦　✦

myrrh .... 4 drops
chamomile .... 4 drops
orange .... 4 drops
lemon .... 3 drops
carrier oil .... 1 teaspoon (5 ml)

✦　✦　✦

geranium .... 4 drops
cedarwood .... 3 drops
marjoram .... 3 drops
clary sage .... 2 drops
benzoin .... 2 drops
celery .... 1 drop
carrier oil .... 1 teaspoon (5 ml)

petitgrain .... 5 drops
lemon .... 4 drops
fennel .... 3 drops
cinnamon .... 2 drops
melissa .... 1 drop
carrier oil .... 1 teaspoon (5 ml)

✦　✦　✦

marjoram .... 4 drops
petitgrain .... 4 drops
ylang-ylang .... 4 drops
Peru balsam .... 3 drops
carrier oil .... 1 teaspoon (5 ml)

✦　✦　✦

dill .... 3 drops
grapefruit .... 3 drops
allspice .... 3 drops
spruce .... 3 drops
anise .... 3 drops
carrier oil .... 1 teaspoon (5 ml)

✦　✦　✦

lemongrass .... 3 drops
melissa .... 3 drops
allspice .... 3 drops
geranium .... 3 drops
nutmeg .... 3 drops
carrier oil .... 1 teaspoon (5 ml)

FOOT POWDER

Measure the amount of cornstarch, and pour it into a widemouthed glass jar or a spice powder container. Then add the essential oils. Tighten the cap, and let the foot powder sit for a day. Shake before using. Before applying the powder, rub in well at least 5 drops of grapeseed oil with 3 drops of tolu balsam on the bottom of each foot.

peppermint	15 drops		*spearmint*	15 drops
lemon	10 drops		*mandarin*	10 drops
cinnamon	5 drops		*geranium*	5 drops
cornstarch	2 tablespoons (30 ml)		*cornstarch*	2 tablespoons (30 ml)

✦ ✦ ✦

chamomile	20 drops		*grapefruit*	10 drops
clove	5 drops		*spruce*	10 drops
sweet bay	5 drops		*patchouli*	5 drops
cornstarch	2 tablespoons (30 ml)		*lemongrass*	5 drops
			cornstarch	2 tablespoons (30 ml)

✦ ✦ ✦

cypress	10 drops			
eucalyptus	10 drops		*ylang-ylang*	10 drops
clove	5 drops		*ginger*	10 drops
orange	5 drops		*lemon*	10 drops
cornstarch	2 tablespoons (30 ml)		*cornstarch*	2 tablespoons (30 ml)

FURNITURE POLISH

Use this polish on your furniture for a beautiful shine. Combine ingredients and gently polish.

ylang-ylang	10 drops		*jojoba*	1 fluid ounce (30 ml)

Essential oils can strengthen plants and repel insects at the same time.

Fill a container with water; then add the essential oils. Mix well to disperse the oil droplets in the water. Water plants well prior to using one of these solutions. These formulas can be used on a regular basis.

sage	10 drops		*thyme*	10 drops
clove	5 drops		*lavender*	5 drops
water	1 gallon (3.8 L)		*water*	1 gallon (3.8 L)

✦ ✦ ✦

cinnamon	8 drops		*clove*	10 drops
peppermint	7 drops		*sweet bay*	5 drops
water	1 gallon (3.8 L)		*water*	1 gallon (3.8 L)

If your plants or bushes are *already* infested with insects, use one of the stronger solutions below. Fill the mist spray bottle with water, then add the essential oils. Tighten the cap, shake well, and mist the infested plant. Use as minimal an amount as possible. Several applications, a few days apart, may be necessary. These mist sprays can be used on outdoor or indoor plants.

sage	45 drops		*lavender*	50 drops
thyme	45 drops		*fennel*	40 drops
water	4 fluid ounces (120 ml)		*water*	4 fluid ounces (120 ml)

✦ ✦ ✦

peppermint	45 drops		*cinnamon*	50 drops
sweet bay	45 drops		*patchouli*	40 drops
water	4 fluid ounces (120 ml)		*water*	4 fluid ounces (120 ml)

✦ ✦ ✦

clove	45 drops		*coriander*	45 drops
caraway	45 drops		*lavender*	45 drops
water	4 fluid ounces (120 ml)		*water*	4 fluid ounces (120 ml)

HAIR CARE

The condition of the hair is very important to the way you look. Regardless of the style, the hair should be thick, shiny, and soft. These formulas will help promote a natural shine in your hair.

Massage approximately 1 teaspoon into the hair and scalp at one time. It's best to leave on for several hours to allow the oils to penetrate. If you use the formula before bedtime, wrap a towel around your head, and leave on overnight. In the morning, wash your hair twice with a natural shampoo (available in health food stores) and warm water. Use the formula three times a week, until you achieve desired results. It is best to discontinue use of commercial shampoos and harsh chemicals on the hair and scalp to maintain beautiful, shiny hair.

✦ Normal Hair ✦

cedarwood	8 drops	*thyme*	8 drops
rosemary	8 drops	*sage*	6 drops
sweet bay	8 drops	*chamomile*	6 drops
geranium	3 drops	*lavender*	5 drops
jojoba	2 tablespoons (30 ml)	*jojoba*	2 tablespoons (30 ml)

✦ Dry Hair ✦

sandalwood	10 drops	*ginger*	10 drops
bois de rose	10 drops	*bois de rose*	10 drops
palmarosa	5 drops	*lavender*	5 drops
jojoba	2 tablespoons (30 ml)	*sesame*	2 tablespoons (30 ml)

✦ Oily Hair ✦

ylang-ylang	9 drops	*petitgrain*	8 drops
lime	9 drops	*lemon*	8 drops
rosemary	8 drops	*lavender*	8 drops
grapeseed	2 tablespoons (30 ml)	*hazelnut*	2 tablespoons (30 ml)

HAND BATHS

Those people who experience tired and aching hands after a day's work may find relief in one of these hand baths. Select a carrier oil—grapeseed, sweet almond, hazelnut, or sesame—to dilute the essential oils. Add the blend of oils to a basin of warm water and soak your hands for 20 to 30 minutes.

✦ Soothe Aching Muscles ✦

spearmint .... 5 drops		melissa .... 5 drops
palmarosa .... 5 drops		lavender .... 5 drops
geranium .... 5 drops		allspice .... 5 drops
carrier oil .... 1 teaspoon (5 ml)		carrier oil .... 1 teaspoon (5 ml)

✦ ✦ ✦

peppermint .... 4 drops	cypress .... 5 drops
thyme .... 4 drops	cinnamon .... 4 drops
lavender .... 4 drops	cajeput .... 4 drops
marjoram .... 3 drops	lemon .... 2 drops
carrier oil .... 1 teaspoon (5 ml)	carrier oil .... 1 teaspoon (5 ml)

✦ ✦ ✦

sweet bay .... 4 drops	geranium .... 5 drops
ginger .... 4 drops	ylang-ylang .... 4 drops
nutmeg .... 4 drops	spearmint .... 4 drops
lavender .... 3 drops	lavender .... 2 drops
carrier oil .... 1 teaspoon (5 ml)	carrier oil .... 1 teaspoon (5 ml)

INSECT BITES

These formulas help to soothe the area of the insect bite and relieve discomfort. Apply the formula to the bite every few hours.

aloe vera gel .... 1 teaspoon (5 ml)
geranium .... 5 drops

✦ ✦ ✦

borage .... 1 teaspoon (5 ml)
juniper berries .... 2 drops
tea tree .... 2 drops
lemon .... 1 drop

✦ ✦ ✦

aloe vera gel .... 1 teaspoon (5 ml)
chamomile .... 5 drops

flaxseed .... 1 teaspoon (5 ml)
sweet basil .... 2 drops
lemon .... 2 drops
marjoram .... 1 drop

✦ ✦ ✦

sesame .... 1 teaspoon (5 ml)
juniper berries .... 2 drops
sweet basil .... 2 drops
lime .... 1 drop

✦ ✦ ✦

aloe vera gel .... 1 teaspoon (5 ml)
lavender .... 5 drops

INSECT REPELLENTS

To deter insects, spray the mist on the exposed areas of the body before going outdoors. Rub jojoba oil into the skin prior to spraying the formula. Spray a minimal amount. Avoid misting on the face; instead, apply this face oil: sandalwood—4 drops, cajeput—4 drops, lavender—2 drops blended in 2 teaspoons of carrier oil.

jojoba .... 100 drops

lavender .... 100 drops

eucalyptus .... 50 drops

lemongrass .... 50 drops

patchouli .... 50 drops

cajeput .... 50 drops

vodka .... 2 fluid ounces (60 ml)

✦ ✦ ✦

jojoba .... 100 drops

geranium .... 100 drops

cedarwood .... 50 drops

sweet bay .... 50 drops

lime .... 50 drops

pine .... 50 drops

vodka .... 2 fluid ounces (60 ml)

jojoba .... 100 drops

cajeput .... 100 drops

lavender .... 100 drops

patchouli .... 100 drops

vodka .... 2 fluid ounces (60 ml)

✦ ✦ ✦

jojoba .... 100 drops

cedarwood .... 75 drops

sandalwood .... 75 drops

lime .... 50 drops

lavender .... 50 drops

geranium .... 50 drops

vodka .... 2 fluid ounces (60 ml)

JACUZZI OILS

Add 5 drops of essential oil per person. If only one person will be in the jacuzzi, increase the amount of oil to 10 drops. Select your favorite oil or choose one of these.

chamomile	eucalyptus	geranium
lavender	myrtle	pine
spearmint	spruce	tea tree

LACTATION

Massage the entire blend into the upper chest. Then rub cornstarch over the same area to absorb any oily residue, since this residue could irritate a baby's tender skin, while nursing.

✦ To Increase Lactation ✦

lemongrass .... 5 drops

sesame .... 1 teaspoon (5 ml)

✦ To Decrease Lactation ✦

peppermint .... 5 drops	*sage* .... 5 drops
grapeseed .... 1 teaspoon (5 ml)	*grapeseed* .... 1 teaspoon (5 ml)

LAUNDRY SCENTS

Put 10 drops of essential oil on a cotton cloth, and place the cloth in the dryer together with the clothes to be scented. Choose any one of these oils.

clove	*lime*	*spearmint*
geranium	*peppermint*	*spruce*
lavender		

Lice are common parasites that infest the hair. These formulas help kill lice and nourish the hair and scalp, as well.

Massage the entire formula vigorously into the hair and scalp before bedtime. Wrap a towel around the head, and leave it on overnight. Repeat nightly until the lice are gone.

geranium	8 drops
rosemary	7 drops
jojoba	1 tablespoon (15 ml)

✦ ✦ ✦

ginger	5 drops
rosemary	5 drops
cajeput	5 drops
walnut	1 tablespoon (15 ml)

thyme	5 drops
rosemary	5 drops
lavender	5 drops
jojoba	1 tablespoon (15 ml)

✦ ✦ ✦

peppermint	5 drops
ginger	5 drops
lavender	5 drops
walnut	1 tablespoon (15 ml)

LIGHT BULB RINGS

The brass ring rests on top of the light bulb and diffuses the desired aroma when the bulb is hot. Choose an oil from one of the scent categories below.

Place five drops of essential oil in the ring before turning on the light. Avoid adding oil when the bulb is hot, since it may shatter. Use only light bulbs that are 60 watts or lower.

Citrus Scent	Floral Scent	Forest Scent	Minty Scent	Spicy Scent
grapefruit	benzoin	eucalyptus	peppermint	allspice
lemon	jasmine	myrtle	spearmint	caraway
lemongrass	rose	pine		clove
lime	tolu balsam	rosemary		sage
melissa	ylang-ylang	spruce		
neroli				
orange				

MASSAGE OILS

When applying essential oils on the skin, a carrier oil should always be added to the blend. The importance of using a carrier oil is to dilute the essential oils in order to protect the skin from becoming irritated. For *best* results, all massage formulas should be massaged for at least 30 minutes, until all the oil is fully absorbed by the skin. To remove any oil residue after the treatment, rub cornstarch on the area.

   If a specific carrier oil is indicated in the massage formula, be sure to use that carrier. If a carrier oil is not specified, choose one from this list.

sweet almond	*flaxseed*	*jojoba*	*olive*
avocado	*grapeseed*	*kukui nut*	*sesame*
*borage**	*hazelnut*	*macadamia nut*	*walnut*

* Dilute with another carrier oil.

✦ Ache and Pain Relievers ✦

Massage the formula into the specific area(s).

rosemary .... 5 drops		*palmarosa* .... 5 drops	
nutmeg .... 5 drops		*eucalyptus* .... 5 drops	
lavender .... 5 drops		*pine* .... 5 drops	
carrier oil .... 1 tablespoon (15 ml)		*carrier oil* .... 1 tablespoon (15 ml)	

✦ ✦ ✦

✦ ✦ ✦

ginger .... 5 drops		*peppermint* .... 5 drops	
sweet bay .... 5 drops		*allspice* .... 5 drops	
marjoram .... 5 drops		*marjoram* .... 5 drops	
carrier oil .... 1 tablespoon (15 ml)		*carrier oil* .... 1 tablespoon (15 ml)	

MASSAGE OILS

✦ Calming ✦

Massage the blend into the shoulders, back of the neck, and down the back.

petitgrain	6 drops
orange	5 drops
neroli	4 drops
carrier oil	1 tablespoon (15 ml)

✦ ✦ ✦

bois de rose	5 drops
anise	4 drops
cajeput	4 drops
sweet basil	2 drops
carrier oil	1 tablespoon (15 ml)

✦ ✦ ✦

petitgrain	5 drops
cedarwood	5 drops
chamomile	5 drops
carrier oil	1 tablespoon (15 ml)

✦ ✦ ✦

sandalwood	5 drops
bois de rose	4 drops
lavender	4 drops
lemongrass	2 drops
carrier oil	1 tablespoon (15 ml)

✦ ✦ ✦

ylang-ylang	5 drops
orange	5 drops
petitgrain	5 drops
carrier oil	1 tablespoon (15 ml)

✦ ✦ ✦

myrrh	4 drops
mandarin	4 drops
spruce	4 drops
neroli	3 drops
carrier oil	1 tablespoon (15 ml)

✦ ✦ ✦

chamomile	5 drops
bergamot	5 drops
lavender	5 drops
carrier oil	1 tablespoon (15 ml)

✦ ✦ ✦

cedarwood	5 drops
clary sage	4 drops
palmarosa	4 drops
lemon	2 drops
carrier oil	1 tablespoon (15 ml)

✦ ✦ ✦

✦ Calming (continued) ✦

cedarwood	5 drops	*melissa*	5 drops
lemon	5 drops	*allspice*	5 drops
mandarin	5 drops	*benzoin*	5 drops
carrier oil	1 tablespoon (15 ml)	*carrier oil*	1 tablespoon (15 ml)

✦ Cellulite Reduction ✦

Many people have cellulite. With the use of these cellulite-reducing blends and a wholesome diet, reducing weight and inches is feasible. Massage the formula into the cellulite area(s). Work deeply into the tissues to help smooth bumpy and dimpled skin.

celery	5 drops	*rosemary*	5 drops
grapefruit	5 drops	*benzoin*	5 drops
cinnamon	5 drops	*fennel*	5 drops
benzoin	5 drops	*lemon*	5 drops
carrier oil	4 teaspoons (20 ml)	*carrier oil*	4 teaspoons (20 ml)

✦ ✦ ✦

pine	4 drops	*cypress*	5 drops
juniper berries	4 drops	*benzoin*	5 drops
fennel	4 drops	*rosemary*	5 drops
lime	4 drops	*sweet basil*	4 drops
thyme	4 drops	*carrier oil*	4 teaspoons (20 ml)
carrier oil	4 teaspoons (20 ml)		

✦ ✦ ✦

✦ ✦ ✦

rosemary .... 4 drops	geranium .... 5 drops
celery .... 4 drops	celery .... 5 drops
cypress .... 4 drops	lime .... 5 drops
pine .... 3 drops	benzoin .... 3 drops
cinnamon .... 3 drops	black pepper .... 2 drops
thyme .... 2 drops	carrier oil .... 4 teaspoons (20 ml)
carrier oil .... 4 teaspoons (20 ml)	

✦ ✦ ✦

	grapefruit .... 5 drops
fennel .... 5 drops	pine .... 5 drops
pine .... 5 drops	cinnamon .... 5 drops
thyme .... 5 drops	fennel .... 3 drops
benzoin .... 5 drops	cypress .... 2 drops
carrier oil .... 4 teaspoons (20 ml)	carrier oil .... 4 teaspoons (20 ml)

✦ Communication Enhancement ✦

Lack of communication may be the first indication of a troubled relationship. These formulas help encourage the flow of feelings that have been repressed.

Apply the formula to the upper chest, back of the neck, and shoulders.

frankincense .... 5 drops	frankincense .... 5 drops
benzoin .... 5 drops	clary sage .... 5 drops
geranium .... 5 drops	sandalwood .... 5 drops
carrier oil .... 1 tablespoon (15 ml)	carrier oil .... 1 tablespoon (15 ml)

✦ ✦ ✦

spruce .... 5 drops	ylang-ylang .... 5 drops
pine .... 5 drops	pine .... 5 drops
clary sage .... 5 drops	frankincense .... 5 drops
carrier oil .... 1 tablespoon (15 ml)	carrier oil .... 1 tablespoon (15 ml)

✦ ✦ ✦   ✦ ✦ ✦

✦ Communication Enhancement (continued) ✦

lemon	5 drops		grapefruit	6 drops
sandalwood	5 drops		spruce	5 drops
clary sage	5 drops		patchouli	4 drops
carrier oil	1 tablespoon (15 ml)		carrier oil	1 tablespoon (15 ml)

✦ Fatigue Relief ✦

Fatigue can result from strenuous physical or mental work, stress, or not getting a restful sleep. Try one of the Sleep Restfully formulas before bedtime. Then, in the morning, apply one of these formulas to energize you.

Massage the blend into the upper chest, back of the neck, shoulders, and down the back.

lime	5 drops		grapefruit	6 drops
cumin	5 drops		palmarosa	5 drops
clove	5 drops		thyme	4 drops
carrier oil	1 tablespoon (15 ml)		carrier oil	1 tablespoon (15 ml)

✦ ✦ ✦

spearmint	6 drops		bergamot	5 drops
pine	5 drops		lemon	5 drops
ginger	4 drops		cumin	5 drops
carrier oil	1 tablespoon (15 ml)		carrier oil	1 tablespoon (15 ml)

✦ ✦ ✦

rosemary	5 drops		peppermint	6 drops
melissa	5 drops		rosemary	5 drops
cumin	5 drops		grapefruit	4 drops
carrier oil	1 tablespoon (15 ml)		carrier oil	1 tablespoon (15 ml)

✦ Foot Rejuvenator ✦

To rejuvenate tired and aching feet, try these formulas. Massage the formula from the bottoms of the feet up to the calves.

cajeput	4 drops
lime	4 drops
rosemary	4 drops
cypress	4 drops
pine	4 drops
carrier oil	4 teaspoons (20 ml)

✦ ✦ ✦

lavender	5 drops
palmarosa	4 drops
allspice	4 drops
lemon	4 drops
patchouli	3 drops
carrier oil	4 teaspoons (20 ml)

✦ ✦ ✦

grapefruit	4 drops
geranium	4 drops
myrtle	3 drops
lime	3 drops
palmarosa	3 drops
thyme	3 drops
carrier oil	4 teaspoons (20 ml)

lavender	4 drops
cajeput	4 drops
coriander	4 drops
cubeb	4 drops
eucalyptus	4 drops
carrier oil	4 teaspoons (20 ml)

✦ ✦ ✦

spearmint	4 drops
ginger	4 drops
petitgrain	4 drops
cypress	3 drops
spruce	3 drops
eucalyptus	2 drops
carrier oil	4 teaspoons (20 ml)

✦ ✦ ✦

peppermint	5 drops
lemon	4 drops
tea tree	4 drops
sage	4 drops
spruce	3 drops
carrier oil	4 teaspoons (20 ml)

✦ Hand Rejuvenator ✦

Massage the formula into both hands, from the fingers to the shoulders.

allspice .... 5 drops	melissa .... 5 drops
rosemary .... 5 drops	cypress .... 5 drops
peppermint .... 5 drops	peppermint .... 5 drops
lavender .... 5 drops	cinnamon .... 5 drops
carrier oil .... 4 teaspoons (20 ml)	carrier oil .... 4 teaspoons (20 ml)

✦ ✦ ✦

grapefruit .... 5 drops	lavender .... 5 drops
black pepper .... 5 drops	nutmeg .... 4 drops
spearmint .... 5 drops	sweet basil .... 3 drops
ginger .... 5 drops	lemon .... 3 drops
carrier oil .... 4 teaspoons (20 ml)	juniper berries .... 3 drops
	allspice .... 2 drops
	carrier oil .... 4 teaspoons (20 ml)

✦ ✦ ✦

lime .... 5 drops	geranium .... 5 drops
thyme .... 5 drops	grapefruit .... 5 drops
eucalyptus .... 5 drops	sweet bay .... 5 drops
cajeput .... 5 drops	black pepper .... 5 drops
carrier oil .... 4 teaspoons (20 ml)	carrier oil .... 4 teaspoons (20 ml)

✦ Mood Uplifting ✦

Massage the formula into the upper chest, back of the neck, and shoulders.

palmarosa .... 4 drops	ylang-ylang .... 5 drops
ylang-ylang .... 4 drops	ginger .... 4 drops
orange .... 4 drops	patchouli .... 3 drops
lime .... 3 drops	bois de rose .... 3 drops
carrier oil .... 1 tablespoon (15 ml)	carrier oil .... 1 tablespoon (15 ml)

✦ ✦ ✦

melissa .... 5 drops	rose .... 5 drops
jasmine .... 5 drops	geranium .... 4 drops
lemon .... 5 drops	patchouli .... 4 drops
carrier oil .... 1 tablespoon (15 ml)	clove .... 2 drops
	carrier oil .... 1 tablespoon (15 ml)

✦ ✦ ✦

lemongrass .... 5 drops	
geranium .... 5 drops	ylang-ylang .... 5 drops
sweet basil .... 3 drops	caraway .... 4 drops
lime .... 2 drops	sandalwood .... 4 drops
carrier oil .... 1 tablespoon (15 ml)	cardamom .... 2 drops
	carrier oil .... 1 tablespoon (15 ml)

✦ ✦ ✦

peppermint .... 5 drops	
thyme .... 4 drops	frankincense .... 5 drops
grapefruit .... 4 drops	ginger .... 5 drops
cypress .... 2 drops	grapefruit .... 5 drops
carrier oil .... 1 tablespoon (15 ml)	carrier oil .... 1 tablespoon (15 ml)

MASSAGE OILS

✦ Muscle Relaxers ✦

Massage the formula into tight muscles and the surrounding areas.

ginger	10 drops
cypress	10 drops
juniper berries	5 drops
black pepper	5 drops
sesame	2 tablespoons (30 ml)

✦ ✦ ✦

ginger	15 drops
ylang-ylang	9 drops
black pepper	6 drops
sesame	2 tablespoons (30 ml)

Peru balsam	9 drops
thyme	8 drops
sweet bay	7 drops
marjoram	6 drops
sesame	2 tablespoons (30 ml)

✦ ✦ ✦

geranium	10 drops
ginger	10 drops
cypress	5 drops
juniper berries	5 drops
sesame	2 tablespoons (30 ml)

MASSAGE OILS

✦ For Muscle Soreness ✦

Massage the formula into the specific muscles.

ylang-ylang .... 5 drops	sweet bay .... 4 drops
ginger .... 5 drops	rosemary .... 4 drops
nutmeg .... 3 drops	eucalyptus .... 4 drops
rosemary .... 2 drops	ylang-ylang .... 3 drops
carrier oil .... 1 tablespoon (15 ml)	carrier oil .... 1 tablespoon (15 ml)

✦ ✦ ✦

ylang-ylang .... 4 drops	cinnamon .... 4 drops
peppermint .... 4 drops	geranium .... 3 drops
thyme .... 3 drops	juniper berries .... 3 drops
ginger .... 3 drops	lavender .... 3 drops
lemon .... 1 drop	peppermint .... 2 drops
carrier oil .... 1 tablespoon (15 ml)	carrier oil .... 1 tablespoon (15 ml)

✦ ✦ ✦

allspice .... 5 drops	grapefruit .... 5 drops
cinnamon .... 4 drops	rose .... 5 drops
cajeput .... 3 drops	tea tree .... 3 drops
chamomile .... 3 drops	spearmint .... 2 drops
carrier oil .... 1 tablespoon (15 ml)	carrier oil .... 1 tablespoon (15 ml)

✦ ✦ ✦

geranium .... 5 drops	spearmint .... 5 drops
peppermint .... 4 drops	sweet bay .... 4 drops
marjoram .... 3 drops	benzoin .... 4 drops
allspice .... 3 drops	lavender .... 2 drops
carrier oil .... 1 tablespoon (15 ml)	carrier oil .... 1 tablespoon (15 ml)

✦ Physical Endurance ✦

For centuries, humans have sought ways to increase physical strength and endurance. Whether in hand-to-hand combat or competitive sports, it was advantageous to be as strong as possible.

A simple before-and-after test can be performed by first completing an exercise, such as push-ups, and recording the number accomplished. Then select one of these physical endurance formulas and massage the blend into the specific muscles that were exerted during the exercise. Wait an hour, repeat the exercise, and record the results. After 7 days of daily application, there should be noticeable improvement.

ginger	6 drops
thyme	5 drops
peppermint	5 drops
celery	5 drops
grapefruit	5 drops
lemon	4 drops
grapeseed	2 tablespoons (30 ml)

✦ ✦ ✦

rosemary	5 drops
geranium	5 drops
grapefruit	5 drops
celery	5 drops
rose	5 drops
bois de rose	5 drops
grapeseed	2 tablespoons (30 ml)

✦ ✦ ✦

grapefruit	7 drops
cajeput	6 drops
palmarosa	6 drops
rosemary	6 drops
thyme	5 drops
sesame	2 tablespoons (30 ml)

✦ ✦ ✦

melissa	5 drops
peppermint	5 drops
palmarosa	5 drops
allspice	5 drops
eucalyptus	4 drops
lime	4 drops
ginger	2 drops
grapeseed	2 tablespoons (30 ml)

✦ ✦ ✦

ginger	5 drops		palmarosa	6 drops
myrtle	5 drops		rose	6 drops
tea tree	5 drops		eucalyptus	5 drops
rose	5 drops		cypress	5 drops
thyme	5 drops		spearmint	5 drops
bois de rose	5 drops		pine	3 drops
grapeseed	2 tablespoons (30 ml)		grapeseed	2 tablespoons (30 ml)

◆ ◆ ◆

spearmint	6 drops		melissa	5 drops
cinnamon	5 drops		bois de rose	5 drops
celery	5 drops		geranium	5 drops
bois de rose	5 drops		palmarosa	5 drops
allspice	5 drops		spearmint	5 drops
lime	4 drops		allspice	5 drops
borage	1 tablespoon (15 ml)		sesame	2 tablespoons (30 ml)
grapeseed	1 tablespoon (15 ml)			

✦ Pre-Event Stress ✦

For those who experience uneasiness or nervous tension before attending an important event or performing, these formulas will help overcome anxiety.

Massage the formula into the back of the neck and the shoulders. Use twice—6 hours apart—before the event.

rose	5 drops		sweet bay	5 drops
neroli	5 drops		palmarosa	5 drops
spruce	4 drops		bergamot	4 drops
rosemary	3 drops		nutmeg	3 drops
bois de rose	3 drops		lavender	2 drops
carrier oil	4 teaspoons (20 ml)		carrier oil	4 teaspoons (20 ml)

◆ ◆ ◆   ◆ ◆ ◆

✦ Pre-Event Stress (continued) ✦

cypress	5 drops		geranium	5 drops
eucalyptus	4 drops		coriander	3 drops
geranium	4 drops		palmarosa	3 drops
chamomile	3 drops		lime	3 drops
benzoin	3 drops		nutmeg	3 drops
lemon	1 drop		lavender	3 drops
carrier oil	4 teaspoons (20 ml)		carrier oil	4 teaspoons (20 ml)

✦ ✦ ✦

melissa	5 drops		allspice	5 drops
chamomile	4 drops		basil	3 drops
fennel	4 drops		lime	3 drops
cinnamon	3 drops		grapefruit	3 drops
grapefruit	3 drops		cinnamon	3 drops
lavender	1 drop		cubeb	3 drops
carrier oil	4 teaspoons (20 ml)		carrier oil	4 teaspoons (20 ml)

✦ ✦ ✦

geranium	5 drops		bois de rose	5 drops
melissa	5 drops		bergamot	5 drops
petitgrain	5 drops		nutmeg	4 drops
cypress	5 drops		mandarin	4 drops
carrier oil	4 teaspoons(20 ml)		melissa	2 drops
			carrier oil	4 teaspoons (20 ml)

✦ Pre-Game Massage ✦

When you compete in sports, it is important to be at your best. Massaging the muscles before the game will help improve your performance.

sweet bay	5 drops
allspice	4 drops
palmarosa	4 drops
grapefruit	4 drops
eucalyptus	3 drops
borage	2 teaspoons (10 ml)
flaxseed	2 teaspoons (10 ml)

✦ ✦ ✦

bois de rose	5 drops
cumin	5 drops
peppermint	5 drops
black pepper	3 drops
lemon	2 drops
sesame	2 teaspoons (10 ml)
grapeseed	2 teaspoons (10 ml)

✦ ✦ ✦

melissa	5 drops
lime	5 drops
cypress	4 drops
cajeput	4 drops
ginger	2 drops
sesame	4 teaspoons (20 ml)

ginger	5 drops
palmarosa	5 drops
geranium	4 drops
bois de rose	4 drops
allspice	2 drops
sesame	4 teaspoons (20 ml)

✦ ✦ ✦

grapefruit	5 drops
peppermint	5 drops
thyme	4 drops
nutmeg	3 drops
black pepper	3 drops
flaxseed	2 teaspoons (10 ml)
borage	2 teaspoons (10 ml)

✦ ✦ ✦

allspice	5 drops
eucalyptus	5 drops
ginger	3 drops
black pepper	3 drops
lavender	2 drops
spearmint	2 drops
carrier oil	4 teaspoons (20 ml)

✦ Premenstrual Syndrome ✦

Before the onset of premenstrual syndrome, massage the blend into the lower back at least once a day.

chamomile .... 7 drops	*rose* .... 10 drops
geranium .... 7 drops	*rosemary* .... 5 drops
lavender .... 7 drops	*grapefruit* .... 5 drops
bois de rose .... 5 drops	*ylang-ylang* .... 5 drops
clary sage .... 4 drops	*cypress* .... 5 drops
borage .... 1 tablespoon (15 ml)	*evening primrose* .... 1 tablespoon (15 ml)
jojoba .... 1 tablespoon (15 ml)	*jojoba* .... 1 tablespoon (15 ml)

✦ ✦ ✦

chamomile .... 5 drops	*caraway* .... 5 drops
allspice .... 5 drops	*sandalwood* .... 5 drops
melissa .... 5 drops	*ylang-ylang* .... 5 drops
bois de rose .... 5 drops	*cumin* .... 5 drops
cypress .... 5 drops	*thyme* .... 5 drops
ginger .... 5 drops	*chamomile* .... 5 drops
sesame .... 1 tablespoon (15 ml)	*evening primrose* .... 1 tablespoon (15 ml)
borage .... 1 tablespoon (15 ml)	*flaxseed* .... 1 tablespoon (15 ml)

✦ ✦ ✦

rose .... 10 drops	*allspice* .... 7 drops
ylang-ylang .... 8 drops	*neroli* .... 7 drops
bergamot .... 7 drops	*geranium* .... 7 drops
geranium .... 5 drops	*petitgrain* .... 5 drops
sesame .... 2 tablespoons (30 ml)	*benzoin* .... 4 drops
	evening primrose .... 1 tablespoon (15 ml)
	jojoba .... 1 tablespoon (15 ml)

✦ ✦ ✦

✦ ✦ ✦

ylang-ylang	8 drops		geranium	8 drops
sandalwood	8 drops		bergamot	7 drops
caraway	5 drops		melissa	6 drops
clary sage	5 drops		fennel	4 drops
anise	4 drops		palmarosa	4 drops
sesame	2 tablespoons (30 ml)		flaxseed	2 tablespoons (30 ml)

✦ Refreshing ✦

Massage the formula into the back of the neck, the shoulders, and along the back.

spearmint	5 drops		pine	5 drops
sweet basil	3 drops		geranium	5 drops
lime	3 drops		grapefruit	4 drops
rosemary	3 drops		peppermint	3 drops
eucalyptus	3 drops		petitgrain	3 drops
bergamot	3 drops		carrier oil	4 teaspoons (20 ml)
carrier oil	4 teaspoons (20 ml)			

✦ ✦ ✦

grapefruit	5 drops		peppermint	5 drops
lemon	5 drops		rosemary	4 drops
eucalyptus	5 drops		clove	3 drops
cajeput	3 drops		lime	3 drops
bois de rose	2 drops		lavender	3 drops
carrier oil	4 teaspoons (20 ml)		sweet basil	2 drops
			carrier oil	4 teaspoons (20 ml)

✦ Romance ✦

Make every evening special for you and your partner with your loving touch. For those precious moments, it is important to leave behind the pressures of the world, focus on each other, and enjoy the evening together.

Massage the formula into the back, neck, and shoulders of your partner until the oil is fully absorbed in the skin. This treatment should be mutually reciprocated for best results.

ylang-ylang .... 5 drops
patchouli .... 3 drops
clove .... 3 drops
orange .... 3 drops
clary sage .... 1 drop
carrier oil .... 1 tablespoon (15 ml)

✦ ✦ ✦

bois de rose .... 5 drops
cedarwood .... 5 drops
jasmine .... 5 drops
carrier oil .... 1 tablespoon (15 ml)

✦ ✦ ✦

rose .... 5 drops
anise .... 4 drops
benzoin .... 4 drops
orange .... 2 drops
carrier oil .... 1 tablespoon (15 ml)

✦ ✦ ✦

palmarosa .... 5 drops
ylang-ylang .... 5 drops
patchouli .... 5 drops
carrier oil .... 1 tablespoon (15 ml)

✦ ✦ ✦

ylang-ylang .... 4 drops
clary sage .... 4 drops
palmarosa .... 4 drops
sandalwood .... 3 drops
carrier oil .... 1 tablespoon (15 ml)

✦ ✦ ✦

geranium .... 4 drops
neroli .... 4 drops
clary sage .... 3 drops
palmarosa .... 3 drops
anise .... 1 drop
carrier oil .... 1 tablespoon (15 ml)

✦ ✦ ✦

ylang-ylang .... 5 drops	sandalwood .... 5 drops
benzoin .... 5 drops	ylang-ylang .... 5 drops
nutmeg .... 3 drops	black pepper .... 3 drops
spruce .... 2 drops	ginger .... 2 drops
carrier oil .... 1 tablespoon (15 ml)	carrier oil .... 1 tablespoon (15 ml)

✦ Sleep Restfully ✦

Before going to sleep, massage the blend into the upper chest, back of the neck, shoulders, and along the back. Do not drive or do anything that requires full attention after applying these formulas. Good night!

celery .... 4 drops
lavender .... 4 drops
nutmeg .... 4 drops
lemon .... 3 drops
carrier oil .... 1 tablespoon (15 ml)

✦ ✦ ✦

petitgrain .... 5 drops
rose .... 5 drops
myrtle .... 3 drops
benzoin .... 2 drops
carrier oil .... 1 tablespoon (15 ml)

✦ ✦ ✦

mandarin .... 4 drops
lavender .... 4 drops
nutmeg .... 3 drops
lemon .... 2 drops
dill .... 2 drops
carrier oil .... 1 tablespoon (15 ml)

✦ ✦ ✦

sandalwood .... 4 drops
marjoram .... 3 drops
bois de rose .... 3 drops
chamomile .... 3 drops
celery .... 2 drops
carrier oil .... 1 tablespoon (15 ml)

✦ ✦ ✦

benzoin .... 5 drops
sweet basil .... 3 drops
celery .... 3 drops
sandalwood .... 3 drops
lemon .... 1 drop
carrier oil .... 1 tablespoon (15 ml)

✦ ✦ ✦

petitgrain .... 4 drops
lavender .... 4 drops
lemongrass .... 4 drops
sweet bay .... 3 drops
carrier oil .... 1 tablespoon (15 ml)

✦ ✦ ✦

✦ Sleep Restfully (continued) ✦

Peru balsam	4 drops		spruce	4 drops
celery	4 drops		marjoram	4 drops
orange	4 drops		melissa	4 drops
sweet basil	3 drops		allspice	3 drops
carrier oil	1 tablespoon (15 ml)		carrier oil	1 tablespoon (15 ml)

✦ ✦ ✦

orange	4 drops		dill	4 drops
anise	3 drops		celery	4 drops
cedarwood	3 drops		cedarwood	4 drops
neroli	3 drops		petitgrain	3 drops
chamomile	2 drops		carrier oil	1 tablespoon (15 ml)
carrier oil	1 tablespoon (15 ml)			

✦ Snoring Remedy ✦

Massage the formula into the upper chest, back of the neck, shoulders, and along the back before going to bed.

bois de rose	4 drops		cajeput	4 drops
geranium	4 drops		myrtle	4 drops
sweet basil	3 drops		marjoram	3 drops
allspice	3 drops		chamomile	3 drops
anise	3 drops		petitgrain	3 drops
lemongrass	3 drops		lavender	3 drops
carrier oil	4 teaspoons (20 ml)		carrier oil	4 teaspoons (20 ml)

✦ ✦ ✦

cubeb .... 4 drops	lavender .... 5 drops
sweet bay .... 4 drops	marjoram .... 4 drops
marjoram .... 4 drops	myrtle .... 4 drops
lavender .... 4 drops	geranium .... 4 drops
sandalwood .... 4 drops	cajeput .... 3 drops
carrier oil .... 4 teaspoons (20 ml)	carrier oil .... 4 teaspoons (20 ml)

✦ ✦ ✦

chamomile .... 4 drops	rose .... 5 drops
geranium .... 4 drops	myrtle .... 4 drops
tea tree .... 3 drops	marjoram .... 3 drops
lavender .... 3 drops	clary sage .... 3 drops
grapefruit .... 3 drops	chamomile .... 3 drops
cubeb .... 3 drops	eucalyptus .... 2 drops
carrier oil .... 4 teaspoons (20 ml)	carrier oil .... 4 teaspoons (20 ml)

✦ For Sprains ✦

Massage the formula into the sprained area. Several applications may be necessary throughout the day, until the painful area feels better.

cypress .... 5 drops	chamomile .... 5 drops
rose .... 5 drops	peppermint .... 5 drops
lemongrass .... 5 drops	cypress .... 5 drops
carrier oil .... 1 tablespoon (15 ml)	carrier oil .... 1 tablespoon (15 ml)

✦ ✦ ✦

cajeput .... 5 drops	celery .... 5 drops
lavender .... 4 drops	lemongrass .... 5 drops
celery .... 4 drops	spearmint .... 3 drops
cypress .... 2 drops	eucalyptus .... 2 drops
carrier oil .... 1 tablespoon (15 ml)	carrier oil .... 1 tablespoon (15 ml)

✦ ✦ ✦

✦ For Sprains (continued) ✦

lavender .... 5 drops	spearmint .... 5 drops
peppermint .... 5 drops	marjoram .... 3 drops
ginger .... 5 drops	cinnamon .... 3 drops
carrier oil .... 1 tablespoon (15 ml)	lemongrass .... 3 drops
	pine .... 1 drop
	carrier oil .... 1 tablespoon (15 ml)

✦ Stress Relievers ✦

Massage the formula into the back of the neck, shoulders, along the back, especially the midsection, and any other tense areas.

melissa .... 5 drops	bergamot .... 5 drops
lavender .... 5 drops	mandarin .... 4 drops
chamomile .... 5 drops	lavender .... 4 drops
nutmeg .... 3 drops	nutmeg .... 4 drops
benzoin .... 2 drops	lemongrass .... 3 drops
carrier oil .... 4 teaspoons (20 ml)	carrier oil .... 4 teaspoons (20 ml)

✦ ✦ ✦

petitgrain .... 5 drops	allspice .... 5 drops
chamomile .... 5 drops	dill .... 4 drops
marjoram .... 3 drops	fennel .... 3 drops
grapefruit .... 3 drops	cinnamon .... 3 drops
bois de rose .... 2 drops	mandarin .... 3 drops
allspice .... 2 drops	marjoram .... 3 drops
carrier oil .... 4 teaspoons (20 ml)	carrier oil .... 4 teaspoons (20 ml)

✦ ✦ ✦

orange .... 5 drops

bois de rose .... 5 drops

petitgrain .... 5 drops

sandalwood .... 5 drops

carrier oil .... 4 teaspoons (20 ml)

✦ ✦ ✦

allspice .... 5 drops

petitgrain .... 5 drops

cypress .... 5 drops

mandarin .... 5 drops

carrier oil .... 4 teaspoons (20 ml)

benzoin .... 5 drops

petitgrain .... 5 drops

eucalyptus .... 5 drops

sandalwood .... 5 drops

carrier oil .... 4 teaspoons (20 ml)

✦ ✦ ✦

cedarwood .... 4 drops

nutmeg .... 4 drops

chamomile .... 4 drops

melissa .... 4 drops

celery .... 4 drops

carrier oil .... 4 teaspoons (20 ml)

✦ Studying for Exams ✦

To increase alertness and retention of information when you are studying, use one of these formulas.

Before studying, massage the formula into the back of the neck and shoulders. On the day of the exam, apply on a cotton ball the same essential oils used when studying. Place the cotton ball inside a plastic bag and seal tightly. Bring the bag with you and inhale the aromas deeply before and during the exam.

ginger .... 6 drops

grapefruit .... 5 drops

juniper berries .... 4 drops

carrier oil .... 1 tablespoon (15 ml)

✦ ✦ ✦

peppermint .... 5 drops

clove .... 5 drops

thyme .... 5 drops

carrier oil .... 1 tablespoon (15 ml)

✦ ✦ ✦

sweet basil .... 5 drops

rosemary .... 5 drops

lemon .... 5 drops

carrier oil .... 1 tablespoon (15 ml)

✦ ✦ ✦

cypress .... 5 drops

rosemary .... 5 drops

coriander .... 5 drops

carrier oil .... 1 tablespoon (15 ml)

✦ ✦ ✦

✦ Studying for Exams (continued) ✦

bergamot .... 5 drops

peppermint .... 5 drops

cypress .... 3 drops

cinnamon .... 2 drops

carrier oil .... 1 tablespoon (15 ml)

✦ ✦ ✦

grapefruit .... 6 drops

petitgrain .... 5 drops

black pepper .... 4 drops

carrier oil .... 1 tablespoon (15 ml)

✦ ✦ ✦

lime .... 5 drops

clove .... 5 drops

rosemary .... 3 drops

spearmint .... 2 drops

carrier oil .... 1 tablespoon (15 ml)

lime .... 5 drops

rosemary .... 5 drops

spearmint .... 5 drops

carrier oil .... 1 tablespoon (15 ml)

✦ ✦ ✦

lemon .... 5 drops

peppermint .... 5 drops

sweet basil .... 3 drops

cypress .... 2 drops

carrier oil .... 1 tablespoon (15 ml)

✦ ✦ ✦

grapefruit .... 5 drops

bergamot .... 5 drops

clove .... 5 drops

carrier oil .... 1 tablespoon (15 ml)

MASSAGE OILS

✦ Travel Comfortably ✦

Many people experience discomfort while travelling. These formulas will help you have an enjoyable trip. Massage the formula into the abdomen, chest, back, and shoulders, 1 hour before travelling.

sweet bay .... 5 drops	bois de rose .... 5 drops
peppermint .... 4 drops	ginger .... 4 drops
chamomile .... 4 drops	dill .... 4 drops
geranium .... 4 drops	caraway .... 4 drops
ginger .... 3 drops	chamomile .... 3 drops
carrier oil .... 4 teaspoons (20 ml)	carrier oil .... 4 teaspoons (20 ml)

✦ ✦ ✦

allspice .... 5 drops	melissa .... 5 drops
vetiver .... 5 drops	cypress .... 5 drops
lavender .... 5 drops	petitgrain .... 5 drops
caraway .... 5 drops	lemongrass .... 5 drops
carrier oil .... 4 teaspoons (20 ml)	carrier oil .... 4 teaspoons (20 ml)

✦ ✦ ✦

chamomile .... 5 drops	mandarin .... 5 drops
ginger .... 4 drops	lavender .... 4 drops
sandalwood .... 4 drops	juniper berries .... 4 drops
celery .... 4 drops	allspice .... 4 drops
nutmeg .... 3 drops	geranium .... 3 drops
carrier oil .... 4 teaspoons (20 ml)	carrier oil .... 4 teaspoons (20 ml)

✦ ✦ ✦

✦ Travel Comfortably (continued) ✦

palmarosa	4 drops	*grapefruit*	5 drops
cubeb	4 drops	*lavender*	5 drops
allspice	4 drops	*sweet basil*	3 drops
cinnamon	4 drops	*thyme*	3 drops
spearmint	4 drops	*clove*	3 drops
carrier oil	4 teaspoons (20 ml)	*geranium*	1 drop
		carrier oil	4 teaspoons (20 ml)

Essential oils not only produce a wonderfully scented atmosphere, but they provide a multitude of desirable effects. Refer to Air Fresheners for directions to prepare sprays in this section. For best results, mist over your head about 10 times. With every 2 to 3 sprays, stop and inhale deeply. Be sure to close your eyes to avoid any eye irritation.

✦ Alertness ✦

Many people have difficulty getting going in the morning. To help revitalize the body and feel rejuvenated, use these mists.

peppermint .... 85 drops

ginger .... 40 drops

grapefruit .... 35 drops

sweet basil .... 15 drops

pure water .... 4 fluid ounces (120 ml)

peppermint .... 60 drops

rosemary .... 40 drops

cypress .... 40 drops

clove .... 35 drops

pure water .... 4 fluid ounces (120 ml)

✦ ✦ ✦

lime .... 70 drops

peppermint .... 45 drops

cypress .... 30 drops

cinnamon .... 30 drops

pure water .... 4 fluid ounces (120 ml)

✦ ✦ ✦

eucalyptus .... 30 drops

ginger .... 30 drops

grapefruit .... 30 drops

bergamot .... 30 drops

lime .... 30 drops

rosemary .... 25 drops

pure water .... 4 fluid ounces (120 ml)

MIST SPRAYS

✦ For Alertness When Driving ✦

There are occasions when a person has to drive while in a fatigued state. Many accidents and injuries are caused by drivers who fall asleep at the wheel. If you are *very* tired, do not drive, but if you must drive, spray one of these mists in your car to help you stay awake. Be especially careful not to spray any mist near your eyes.

peppermint	110 drops
cinnamon	35 drops
lime	35 drops
patchouli	20 drops
pure water	4 fluid ounces (120 ml)

✦ ✦ ✦

spearmint	120 drops
cypress	40 drops
lemon	40 drops
pure water	4 fluid ounces (120 ml)

✦ ✦ ✦

lime	75 drops
rosemary	50 drops
clove	45 drops
peppermint	30 drops
pure water	4 fluid ounces (120 ml)

✦ ✦ ✦

rosemary	50 drops
lemon	50 drops
cinnamon	50 drops
geranium	25 drops
cypress	25 drops
pure water	4 fluid ounces (120 ml)

peppermint	80 drops
lime	75 drops
rosemary	45 drops
pure water	4 fluid ounces (120 ml)

✦ ✦ ✦

peppermint	80 drops
thyme	40 drops
rosemary	40 drops
grapefruit	40 drops
pure water	4 fluid ounces (120 ml)

✦ ✦ ✦

pine	60 drops
lemon	60 drops
rosemary	60 drops
sage	20 drops
pure water	4 fluid ounces (120 ml)

✦ ✦ ✦

pine	50 drops
thyme	40 drops
spearmint	40 drops
cumin	25 drops
juniper berries	25 drops
clove	20 drops
pure water	4 fluid ounces (120 ml)

✦ Alertness for Studying ✦

To increase alertness and retention of information, mist numerous times while studying and inhale deeply. On the day of the exam, apply a few drops of each essential oil to a cotton ball from the mist formula used when studying. Place the cotton ball inside a plastic bag and seal tightly. Bring the bag with you, and inhale the aromas deeply before and during the exam.

lime .... 80 drops

rosemary .... 60 drops

ginger .... 20 drops

sweet basil .... 15 drops

pure water .... 4 fluid ounces (120 ml)

✦ ✦ ✦

clove .... 50 drops

pine .... 50 drops

spearmint .... 50 drops

lemon .... 25 drops

pure water .... 4 fluid ounces (120 ml)

✦ ✦ ✦

bergamot .... 40 drops

grapefruit .... 40 drops

peppermint .... 40 drops

juniper berries .... 30 drops

lavender .... 25 drops

pure water .... 4 fluid ounces (120 ml)

lemon .... 70 drops

peppermint .... 45 drops

petitgrain .... 20 drops

clove .... 20 drops

thyme .... 20 drops

pure water .... 4 fluid ounces (120 ml)

✦ ✦ ✦

grapefruit .... 50 drops

clove .... 40 drops

sweet basil .... 30 drops

bergamot .... 30 drops

ginger .... 25 drops

pure water .... 4 fluid ounces (120 ml)

✦ ✦ ✦

spearmint .... 40 drops

lemon .... 40 drops

lavender .... 30 drops

eucalyptus .... 25 drops

rosemary .... 25 drops

sweet basil .... 15 drops

pure water .... 4 fluid ounces (120 ml)

✦ Breathe More Easily during Aerobics, Sports, and Other Exercise ✦

Vigorous exercise strains the respiratory system. Before exercising, spray these mists into the air and breathe deeply to help soothe breathing passages.

peppermint .... 40 drops	*lime* .... 50 drops
eucalyptus .... 40 drops	*pine* .... 40 drops
cajeput .... 40 drops	*tea tree* .... 30 drops
lemon .... 30 drops	*cubeb* .... 30 drops
pure water .... 4 fluid ounces (120 ml)	*pure water* .... 4 fluid ounces (120 ml)

✦ ✦ ✦

spruce .... 40 drops	*tea tree* .... 40 drops
lavender .... 40 drops	*cajeput* .... 40 drops
spearmint .... 35 drops	*lavender* .... 40 drops
eucalyptus .... 35 drops	*myrtle* .... 30 drops
pure water .... 4 fluid ounces (120 ml)	*pure water* .... 4 fluid ounces (120 ml)

✦ ✦ ✦

lime .... 50 drops	*myrtle* .... 40 drops
lavender .... 50 drops	*lemon* .... 40 drops
eucalyptus .... 30 drops	*pine* .... 40 drops
clove .... 20 drops	*lemongrass* .... 30 drops
pure water .... 4 fluid ounces (120 ml)	*pure water* .... 4 fluid ounces (120 ml)

✦ ✦ ✦

✦ ✦ ✦

lavender .... 50 drops

cajeput .... 30 drops

grapefruit .... 20 drops

clove .... 20 drops

spruce .... 20 drops

thyme .... 10 drops

pure water .... 4 fluid ounces (120 ml)

✦ ✦ ✦

pine .... 40 drops

spruce .... 40 drops

grapefruit .... 40 drops

lavender .... 30 drops

pure water .... 4 fluid ounces (120 ml)

myrtle .... 30 drops

cajeput .... 30 drops

eucalyptus .... 30 drops

clove .... 30 drops

lime .... 30 drops

pure water .... 4 fluid ounces (120 ml)

✦ ✦ ✦

peppermint .... 40 drops

rosemary .... 30 drops

lime .... 30 drops

lavender .... 30 drops

marjoram .... 20 drops

pure water .... 4 fluid ounces (120 ml)

✦ Breathe More Easily in Stuffy Rooms ✦

eucalyptus .... 40 drops

lemon .... 40 drops

cypress .... 25 drops

lavender .... 25 drops

grapefruit .... 20 drops

pure water .... 4 fluid ounces (120 ml)

✦ ✦ ✦

spearmint .... 30 drops

pine .... 25 drops

juniper berries .... 20 drops

lemon .... 20 drops

cajeput .... 20 drops

lavender .... 20 drops

myrtle .... 15 drops

pure water .... 4 fluid ounces (120 ml)

rosemary .... 30 drops

geranium .... 30 drops

spruce .... 25 drops

thyme .... 25 drops

lime .... 25 drops

cedarwood .... 15 drops

pure water .... 4 fluid ounces (120 ml)

✦ ✦ ✦

lemongrass .... 30 drops

spruce .... 30 drops

myrtle .... 30 drops

lime .... 30 drops

allspice .... 15 drops

lavender .... 15 drops

pure water .... 4 fluid ounces (120 ml)

✦ Calming ✦

mandarin .... 60 drops

lavender .... 50 drops

bois de rose .... 20 drops

petitgrain .... 20 drops

pure water .... 4 fluid ounces (120 ml)

✦ ✦ ✦

spruce .... 40 drops

lavender .... 40 drops

geranium .... 20 drops

petitgrain .... 20 drops

cedarwood .... 20 drops

lemon .... 10 drops

pure water .... 4 fluid ounces (120 ml)

✦ ✦ ✦

ylang-ylang .... 40 drops

orange .... 30 drops

chamomile .... 25 drops

benzoin .... 25 drops

bois de rose .... 15 drops

melissa .... 15 drops

pure water .... 4 fluid ounces (120 ml)

allspice .... 45 drops

dill .... 25 drops

orange .... 25 drops

Peru balsam .... 25 drops

fennel .... 15 drops

cinnamon .... 15 drops

pure water .... 4 fluid ounces (120 ml)

✦ ✦ ✦

lemongrass .... 35 drops

anise .... 25 drops

allspice .... 25 drops

mandarin .... 25 drops

vetiver .... 20 drops

bergamot .... 20 drops

pure water .... 4 fluid ounces (120 ml)

✦ ✦ ✦

marjoram .... 30 drops

cajeput .... 30 drops

lavender .... 30 drops

petitgrain .... 30 drops

vetiver .... 30 drops

pure water .... 4 fluid ounces (120 ml)

MIST SPRAYS

✦ Calming for Overactive Children ✦

mandarin	40 drops	allspice	30 drops
marjoram	30 drops	chamomile	30 drops
lavender	30 drops	mandarin	30 drops
cedarwood	20 drops	vetiver	30 drops
pure water	4 fluid ounces (120 ml)	pure water	4 fluid ounces (120 ml)

✦ Calming for Overactive Pets ✦

marjoram	60 drops	lavender	50 drops
lavender	40 drops	chamomile	50 drops
orange	20 drops	mandarin	20 drops
pure water	4 fluid ounces (120 ml)	pure water	4 fluid ounces (120 ml)

MIST SPRAYS

✦ Holiday Atmosphere ✦

spruce .... 75 drops

cedarwood .... 25 drops

juniper berries .... 25 drops

pure water .... 4 fluid ounces (120 ml)

✦ ✦ ✦

clove .... 40 drops

cinnamon .... 30 drops

ginger .... 30 drops

orange .... 20 drops

pure water .... 4 fluid ounces (120 ml)

allspice .... 30 drops

dill .... 30 drops

caraway .... 30 drops

clove .... 30 drops

pure water .... 4 fluid ounces (120 ml)

✦ ✦ ✦

cypress .... 40 drops

pine .... 30 drops

eucalyptus .... 30 drops

sandalwood .... 20 drops

pure water .... 4 fluid ounces (120 ml)

✦ Mood Elevation ✦

bergamot .... 60 drops

lime .... 50 drops

geranium .... 20 drops

ylang-ylang .... 20 drops

pure water .... 4 fluid ounces (120 ml)

✦ ✦ ✦

bois de rose .... 50 drops

lemon .... 35 drops

melissa .... 35 drops

geranium .... 30 drops

pure water .... 4 fluid ounces (120 ml)

spearmint .... 60 drops

clove .... 40 drops

grapefruit .... 30 drops

tolu balsam .... 20 drops

pure water .... 4 fluid ounces (120 ml)

✦ ✦ ✦

melissa .... 30 drops

lemongrass .... 30 drops

ylang-ylang .... 30 drops

benzoin .... 20 drops

clove .... 20 drops

cumin .... 20 drops

pure water .... 4 fluid ounces (120 ml)

✦ Premenstrual Syndrome ✦

It has been estimated that nearly 90 percent of women suffer from premenstrual syndrome (PMS) sometime in their lives. The syndrome's effects range from outright violence to mild depression to crying spells. These mists can help elevate the mood and make PMS bearable. Spray many times during the day, and inhale the mist deeply.

bergamot .... 60 drops

geranium .... 60 drops

allspice .... 40 drops

anise .... 30 drops

patchouli .... 10 drops

pure water .... 4 fluid ounces (120 ml)

✦　✦　✦

cypress .... 50 drops

neroli .... 50 drops

bergamot .... 40 drops

orange .... 30 drops

allspice .... 30 drops

pure water .... 4 fluid ounces (120 ml)

✦　✦　✦

lemongrass .... 50 drops

cypress .... 40 drops

fennel .... 30 drops

lavender .... 30 drops

geranium .... 30 drops

caraway .... 20 drops

pure water .... 4 fluid ounces (120 ml)

✦　✦　✦

ylang-ylang .... 35 drops

bergamot .... 35 drops

sandalwood .... 35 drops

lime .... 35 drops

palmarosa .... 30 drops

caraway .... 30 drops

pure water .... 4 fluid ounces (120 ml)

✦　✦　✦

chamomile .... 40 drops

lavender .... 40 drops

lemon .... 40 drops

geranium .... 40 drops

caraway .... 40 drops

pure water .... 4 fluid ounces (120 ml)

✦　✦　✦

neroli .... 40 drops

jasmine .... 30 drops

geranium .... 30 drops

palmarosa .... 30 drops

lime .... 30 drops

allspice .... 30 drops

pure water .... 4 fluid ounces (120 ml)

✦　✦　✦

✦ Premenstrual Syndrome (continued) ✦

geranium	60 drops		petitgrain	60 drops
melissa	60 drops		ylang-ylang	50 drops
grapefruit	40 drops		grapefruit	40 drops
allspice	40 drops		bergamot	30 drops
pure water	4 fluid ounces (120 ml)		fennel	20 drops
			pure water	4 fluid ounces (120 ml)

✦ Refreshing ✦

lime	90 drops		lemon	50 drops
peppermint	50 drops		cypress	50 drops
eucalyptus	10 drops		clove	50 drops
pure water	4 fluid ounces (120 ml)		pure water	4 fluid ounces (120 ml)

✦ ✦ ✦

grapefruit	50 drops		grapefruit	40 drops
lemon	50 drops		petitgrain	40 drops
spearmint	50 drops		peppermint	40 drops
pure water	4 fluid ounces (120 ml)		lime	30 drops
			pure water	4 fluid ounces (120 ml)

MIST SPRAYS

✦ Room Disinfectant ✦

tea tree .... 65 drops

thyme .... 50 drops

eucalyptus .... 35 drops

pure water .... 4 fluid ounces (120 ml)

✦ ✦ ✦

clove .... 75 drops

lavender .... 45 drops

bergamot .... 30 drops

pure water .... 4 fluid ounces (120 ml)

lavender .... 70 drops

allspice .... 40 drops

cinnamon .... 40 drops

pure water .... 4 fluid ounces (120 ml)

✦ ✦ ✦

cinnamon .... 65 drops

patchouli .... 45 drops

lemongrass .... 40 drops

pure water .... 4 fluid ounces (120 ml)

✦ Sauna/Steam Room ✦

Spray the mist away from your body so that when you perspire the spray does not come in contact with your eyes.

eucalyptus .... 30 drops

tea tree .... 30 drops

pine .... 30 drops

lavender .... 30 drops

pure water .... 4 fluid ounces (120 ml)

✦ ✦ ✦

lavender .... 50 drops

cajeput .... 25 drops

spruce .... 25 drops

eucalyptus .... 20 drops

pure water .... 4 fluid ounces (120 ml)

sandalwood .... 60 drops

spearmint .... 60 drops

pure water .... 4 fluid ounces (120 ml)

✦ ✦ ✦

peppermint .... 30 drops

lavender .... 30 drops

cedarwood .... 30 drops

spruce .... 15 drops

eucalyptus .... 15 drops

pure water .... 4 fluid ounces (120 ml)

✦ Snoring Remedy ✦

Mist numerous times before going to sleep and have the snorer inhale deeply. If necessary, mist again during the night to quiet the snorer.

geranium	50 drops
lavender	50 drops
marjoram	50 drops
cedarwood	20 drops
eucalyptus	15 drops
sweet basil	15 drops
pure water	4 fluid ounces (120 ml)

spruce	55 drops
myrtle	45 drops
eucalyptus	30 drops
sweet bay	30 drops
grapefruit	20 drops
marjoram	20 drops
pure water	4 fluid ounces (120 ml)

✦ ✦ ✦

marjoram	60 drops
lemongrass	40 drops
sandalwood	40 drops
myrtle	30 drops
lavender	30 drops
pure water	4 fluid ounces (120 ml)

cajeput	55 drops
allspice	55 drops
lavender	50 drops
grapefruit	20 drops
celery	20 drops
pure water	4 fluid ounces (120 ml)

✦ ✦ ✦

spruce	35 drops
lavender	35 drops
anise	35 drops
sandalwood	35 drops
cubeb	30 drops
lemongrass	30 drops
pure water	4 fluid ounces (120 ml)

dill	40 drops
tea tree	40 drops
orange	30 drops
lemongrass	30 drops
allspice	30 drops
marjoram	30 drops
pure water	4 fluid ounces (120 ml)

✦ Stress Relievers ✦

grapefruit .... 50 drops

mandarin .... 35 drops

allspice .... 35 drops

benzoin .... 30 drops

pure water .... 4 fluid ounces (120 ml)

✦ ✦ ✦

lemon .... 40 drops

sandalwood .... 40 drops

allspice .... 40 drops

bois de rose .... 30 drops

pure water .... 4 fluid ounces (120 ml)

✦ ✦ ✦

melissa .... 70 drops

fennel .... 20 drops

cinnamon .... 20 drops

chamomile .... 20 drops

lavender .... 20 drops

pure water .... 4 fluid ounces (120 ml)

✦ ✦ ✦

allspice .... 50 drops

mandarin .... 50 drops

patchouli .... 20 drops

melissa .... 20 drops

pure water .... 4 fluid ounces (120 ml)

cypress .... 50 drops

lemongrass .... 40 drops

lavender .... 20 drops

clove .... 20 drops

patchouli .... 20 drops

pure water .... 4 fluid ounces (120 ml)

✦ ✦ ✦

petitgrain .... 40 drops

mandarin .... 40 drops

lemongrass .... 40 drops

palmarosa .... 30 drops

pure water .... 4 fluid ounces (120 ml)

✦ ✦ ✦

chamomile .... 60 drops

geranium .... 30 drops

coriander .... 30 drops

lavender .... 30 drops

pure water .... 4 fluid ounces (120 ml)

✦ ✦ ✦

lemon .... 45 drops

dill .... 40 drops

palmarosa .... 35 drops

ylang-ylang .... 30 drops

pure water .... 4 fluid ounces (120 ml)

Mist Sprays

✦ Travel Comfortably ✦

Many people experience discomfort when travelling. These mists will soothe the stomach and help make travelling more enjoyable. Use before and during the trip, as necessary. Inhale deeply.

caraway .... 35 drops
melissa .... 35 drops
lemongrass .... 30 drops
geranium .... 25 drops
lavender .... 25 drops
cinnamon .... 25 drops
pure water .... 4 fluid ounces (120 ml)

✦ ✦ ✦

chamomile .... 35 drops
lemon .... 35 drops
sweet bay .... 30 drops
lavender .... 25 drops
ginger .... 25 drops
cinnamon .... 25 drops
pure water .... 4 fluid ounces (120 ml)

✦ ✦ ✦

spearmint .... 50 drops
melissa .... 45 drops
cinnamon .... 30 drops
lemongrass .... 20 drops
cypress .... 20 drops
allspice .... 10 drops
pure water .... 4 fluid ounces (120 ml)

cypress .... 45 drops
melissa .... 45 drops
chamomile .... 40 drops
fennel .... 25 drops
ginger .... 20 drops
pure water .... 4 fluid ounces (120 ml)

✦ ✦ ✦

ginger .... 30 drops
allspice .... 30 drops
cinnamon .... 30 drops
geranium .... 30 drops
cardamom .... 30 drops
pure water .... 4 fluid ounces (120 ml)

✦ ✦ ✦

caraway .... 45 drops
peppermint .... 30 drops
thyme .... 30 drops
nutmeg .... 20 drops
fennel .... 20 drops
marjoram .... 15 drops
allspice .... 15 drops
pure water .... 4 fluid ounces (120 ml)

MOUTHWASH

For fresh breath, use one of these mouthwashes. Add the essential oils and honey to the water, stir well, and rinse your mouth.

peppermint .... 2 drops
spearmint .... 2 drops
pure water .... 4 fluid ounces (120 ml)
honey .... 1 teaspoon (5 ml)

✦ ✦ ✦

rosemary .... 1 drop
sage .... 1 drop
lemon .... 1 drop
peppermint .... 1 drop
pure water .... 4 fluid ounces (120 ml)
honey .... 1 teaspoon (5 ml)

✦ ✦ ✦

spearmint .... 2 drops
allspice .... 1 drop
mandarin .... 1 drop
pure water .... 4 fluid ounces (120 ml)
honey .... 1 teaspoon (5 ml)

anise .... 2 drops
peppermint .... 1 drop
clove .... 1 drop
pure water .... 4 fluid ounces (120 ml)
honey .... 1 teaspoon (5 ml)

✦ ✦ ✦

allspice .... 2 drops
spearmint .... 1 drop
anise .... 1 drop
pure water .... 4 fluid ounces (120 ml)
honey .... 1 teaspoon (5 ml)

✦ ✦ ✦

lemon .... 2 drops
spearmint .... 2 drops
pure water .... 4 fluid ounces (120 ml)
honey .... 1 teaspoon (5 ml)

POTPOURRI

Making your own potpourri is a wonderful way to scent your home. Gather dried leaves, flowers, and small wood shavings. Crush these plant materials to the desired size. Place 1/2 cup (120 ml) of plant material in a widemouthed glass jar, and add the essential oil formula. Stir the contents well and tighten the lid on the jar. Let the potpourri sit for several days to allow the aroma molecules to be absorbed by the plant material.

✦ Citrus Scent ✦

grapefruit	80 drops	*lime*	100 drops
lemon	50 drops	*orange*	40 drops
clove	50 drops	*cinnamon*	30 drops
benzoin	20 drops	*patchouli*	30 drops

✦ Floral Scent ✦

ylang-ylang	70 drops	*bois de rose*	50 drops
geranium	50 drops	*ylang-ylang*	50 drops
orange	50 drops	*lemon*	30 drops
clove	20 drops	*clove*	30 drops
benzoin	10 drops	*cedarwood*	20 drops

✦ Forest Scent ✦

spruce	100 drops	*eucalyptus*	50 drops
lavender	30 drops	*myrtle*	50 drops
clove	30 drops	*cajeput*	50 drops
rosemary	30 drops	*juniper berries*	30 drops
patchouli	10 drops	*Peru balsam*	20 drops

✦ Minty Scent ✦

spearmint	100 drops	peppermint	110 drops
lemon	50 drops	rosemary	30 drops
petitgrain	20 drops	grapefruit	30 drops
peppermint	20 drops	benzoin	30 drops
benzoin	10 drops		

✦ Spicy Scent ✦

caraway	75 drops	cinnamon	75 drops
clove	75 drops	allspice	75 drops
cumin	30 drops	anise	40 drops
patchouli	20 drops	benzoin	10 drops

PRE-SHAVE

Mix the oils together well, and apply them to the area before shaving.

flaxseed	20 drops	flaxseed	20 drops
lavender	3 drops	bois de rose	2 drops
allspice	1 drop	allspice	1 drop

✦ ✦ ✦

flaxseed	20 drops	flaxseed	20 drops
geranium	2 drops	lavender	2 drops
sweet bay	1 drop	chamomile	1 drop

SKIN CARE

The skin is a very resilient organ of the body. After being scraped, cut, burned, or scratched, it can miraculously heal itself fairly quickly. If treated properly, the skin will show little sign of wear and tear over the years.

Combine all ingredients from the formula to help rejuvenate your skin. Before using, wash your skin thoroughly, then massage in a portion of the formula. Apply daily.

✦ Normal Skin ✦

chamomile .... 10 drops	*lavender* .... 10 drops
bois de rose .... 10 drops	*palmarosa* .... 10 drops
benzoin .... 10 drops	*geranium* .... 10 drops
hazelnut .... 2 tablespoons (30 ml)	*hazelnut* .... 2 tablespoons (30 ml)

✦ ✦ ✦

rose .... 10 drops	*lavender* .... 10 drops
frankincense .... 10 drops	*chamomile* .... 5 drops
jasmine .... 10 drops	*fennel* .... 5 drops
hazelnut .... 2 tablespoons (30 ml)	*benzoin* .... 5 drops
	geranium .... 5 drops
	hazelnut .... 2 tablespoons (30 ml)

✦ Dry Skin ✦

sandalwood .... 10 drops	*patchouli* .... 10 drops
bois de rose .... 10 drops	*palmarosa* .... 10 drops
lavender .... 10 drops	*geranium* .... 10 drops
avocado .... 2 tablespoons (30 ml)	*jojoba* .... 2 tablespoons (30 ml)

✦ ✦ ✦

benzoin .... 10 drops	*chamomile* .... 10 drops
rosemary .... 8 drops	*lavender* .... 10 drops
geranium .... 8 drops	*palmarosa* .... 10 drops
lavender .... 4 drops	*sesame* .... 2 tablespoons (30 ml)
flaxseed .... 2 tablespoons (30 ml)	

SKIN CARE

✦ Oily Skin ✦

ylang-ylang .... 10 drops
lemon .... 10 drops
cypress .... 5 drops
petitgrain .... 5 drops
grapeseed .... 2 tablespoons (30 ml)

✦ ✦ ✦

orange .... 10 drops
lemon .... 10 drops
petitgrain .... 10 drops
grapeseed .... 2 tablespoons (30 ml)

lime .... 15 drops
cypress .... 5 drops
juniper berries .... 5 drops
ylang-ylang .... 5 drops
grapeseed .... 2 tablespoons (30 ml)

✦ ✦ ✦

ylang-ylang .... 8 drops
juniper berries .... 8 drops
orange .... 8 drops
lavender .... 6 drops
grapeseed .... 2 tablespoons (30 ml)

✦ Problem Skin ✦

myrrh .... 10 drops
chamomile .... 10 drops
bois de rose .... 5 drops
lavender .... 5 drops
kukui nut .... 2 tablespoons (30 ml)

✦ ✦ ✦

myrrh .... 15 drops
patchouli .... 10 drops
geranium .... 5 drops
borage .... 1 tablespoon (15 ml)
kukui nut .... 1 tablespoon (15 ml)

✦ ✦ ✦

myrrh .... 10 drops
palmarosa .... 10 drops
frankincense .... 10 drops
borage .... 1 tablespoon (15 ml)
flaxseed .... 1 tablespoon (15 ml)

✦ ✦ ✦

sandalwood .... 10 drops
lavender .... 10 drops
bois de rose .... 10 drops
sesame .... 1 tablespoon (15 ml)
flaxseed .... 1 tablespoon (15 ml)

✦ ✦ ✦

✦ Problem Skin (continued) ✦

lavender .... 20 drops	chamomile .... 15 drops
palmarosa .... 10 drops	bois de rose .... 15 drops
evening primrose .... 1 tablespoon (15 ml)	sesame .... 1 tablespoon (15 ml)
flaxseed .... 1 tablespoon (15 ml)	kukui nut .... 1 tablespoon (15 ml)

✦ ✦ ✦   ✦ ✦ ✦

petitgrain .... 10 drops	myrrh .... 10 drops
benzoin .... 10 drops	lavender .... 10 drops
tea tree .... 10 drops	benzoin .... 10 drops
evening primrose .... 1 tablespoon (15 ml)	borage .... 1 tablespoon (15 ml)
kukui nut .... 1 tablespoon (15 ml)	walnut .... 1 tablespoon (15 ml)

Steam Inhalation

Add 5 to 10 drops of essential oil to a bowl of hot water. Drape a towel over the head, close your eyes, and inhale the vapors. Select from the following oils.

cajeput	lemongrass	peppermint	spearmint
eucalyptus	marjoram	pine	spruce
lavender	myrtle	rosemary	tea tree

Sunburn Relief

Gently apply the formula on the sunburned area, several times a day.

lavender .... 3 drops	*chamomile* .... 3 drops
chamomile .... 2 drops	*geranium* .... 2 drops
aloe vera gel .... 1 teaspoon (5 ml)	*sweet almond* .... 1 teaspoon (5 ml)

✦ ✦ ✦

lavender .... 5 drops	*lavender* .... 5 drops
aloe vera gel .... 1 teaspoon (5 ml)	*avocado* .... 1 teaspoon (5 ml)

Suntan Oil

Many people avoid being outdoors because of the discomfort of getting sunburned. With this jojoba and sesame suntan oil, you will get a wonderful tan. First apply jojoba oil on the entire skin area that will be exposed to the sun. Then rub sesame oil over the same area.

jojoba (to cover area)

sesame (to cover area)

5

ESSENTIAL OILS A TO Z

Allspice (Pimento)

Pimenta officinalis
Scent: Clove
Uses
Warming to the body
Reduces stress
Calming
Relaxes tight muscles
Lessens pain
Promotes restful sleep
Mood uplifting
Vapors help breathing
Improves digestion
Disinfectant

♦ ♦ ♦

Aloe

Aloe vera or *Aloe barbadensis*
Uses
Lessens pain
Healing, moisturizing, rejuvenating for skin
Hydrates dry hair

♦ ♦ ♦

Anise

Pimpinella anisum
Scent: Licorice
Uses
Calming
Lessens pain
Aphrodisiac
Promotes restful sleep
Vapors help breathing
Improves digestion
Increases appetite
Stimulates lactation in nursing mothers

♦ ♦ ♦

(Sweet) Basil

Ocimum basilicum
Scent: Slightly licorice

Uses

Calming

Lessens pain

Promotes restful sleep

Mood uplifting

Helps relieve fatigue

Improves digestion

Stimulates lactation in nursing mothers

Improves mental clarity and memory

Helps reduce cellulite deposits

Purifying effect on the body

Soothes insect bites

✦ ✦ ✦

(Sweet) Bay

Laurus nobilis
Scent: Spicy

Uses

Relaxes tight muscles

Soothes sprains

Lessens pain

Calming

Promotes restful sleep

Vapors help breathing

Improves digestion

Improves mental clarity and memory

Promotes perspiration

Disinfectant

Repels insects

✦ ✦ ✦

Benzoin

Styrax benzoin
Scent: Cinnamon-vanilla

Uses

Warming to the body

Reduces stress

Calming

Helpful for meditation

Relaxes tight muscles

Breaks up congestion

Reduces inflammation

Promotes restful sleep

Mood uplifting

Helps reduce cellulite deposits

Healing to the skin

Preservative in cosmetics

Fixative for perfumes and fragrances

✦ ✦ ✦

Bergamot

Citrus bergamia
Scent: Citrus

Uses

Reduces anxiety, nervous tension, and stress

Balances nervous system

Mood uplifting

Helps relieve fatigue

Disinfectant

✦ ✦ ✦

Bois de Rose (Rosewood)

Aniba rosaeodora
Scent: Slightly rosy

Uses

Relieves nervousness and stress

Calming

Lessens pain

Promotes restful sleep

Mood uplifting

Skin tissue regenerator and moisturizer

✦ ✦ ✦

Cajeput

Melaleuca leucadendron
Scent: Camphor

Uses

Slightly warming to the body

Calming

Relaxes tight muscles

Relieves muscle aches and pains

Promotes restful sleep

Breaks up congestion

Vapors help breathing

Disinfectant

Repels insects

✦ ✦ ✦

Caraway

Carum carvi
Scent: Spicy

Uses

Relieves pain

Vapors help breathing

Improves digestion

Increases appetite

Stimulates lactation in nursing mothers

✦ ✦ ✦

Cardamom

Elettaria cardamomum
Scent: Spicy

Uses

Warming to the body

Relieves pain

Mood uplifting

Improves digestion

Improves mental clarity and memory

✦ ✦ ✦

Cedarwood

Cedrus atlantica
Scent: Woody

Uses

Reduces anxiety and tension

Calming

Relaxes tight muscles

Helpful for meditation

Lessens pain

Promotes restful sleep

Vapors help breathing

Repels insects

◆ ◆ ◆

Celery

Apium graveolens
Scent: Strong celery

Uses

Reduces tension

Calming

Promotes restful sleep

Helps reduce cellulite deposits

Purifying effect on the body

◆ ◆ ◆

Chamomile

Matricaria chamomilla
and
Anthemis nobilis
Scent: Musky

Uses

Reduces stress and tension

Calming

Lessens pain

Promotes restful sleep

Reduces inflammation

Improves digestion

Increases appetite

Healing to the skin

Soothes insect bites

◆ ◆ ◆

Cinnamon Bark and Leaf

Cinnamomum zeylanicum
Scent: Cinnamon

Uses

Warming to the body

Relaxes tight muscles

Lessens pain

Mood uplifting

Aphrodisiac

Helps relieve fatigue

Improves digestion

Increases appetite

Helps reduce cellulite deposits

Disinfectant

Repels insects

◆ ◆ ◆

Clary Sage

Salvia sclarea
Scent: Sweet and spicy
Uses
Reduces stress and tension
Calming
Lessens pain
Promotes restful sleep
Aphrodisiac
Improves digestion
Contains estrogen-like hormone
Encourages communication

✦ ✦ ✦

Clove

Eugenia caryophyllata
Scent: Hot and spicy
Uses
Warming to the body
Relieves pain
Mood uplifting
Helps relieve fatigue
Aphrodisiac
Vapors help breathing
Improves digestion
Improves mental clarity and memory
Disinfectant
Repels insects

✦ ✦ ✦

Coriander

Coriandrum sativum
Scent: Musky
Uses
Relieves pain
Helps relieve fatigue
Improves digestion
Improves mental clarity and memory

✦ ✦ ✦

Cubeb

Piper cubeba
Scent: Peppery
Uses
Relieves pain
Breaks up congestion
Vapors help breathing
Improves digestion

✦ ✦ ✦

Cumin

Cuminum cyminum
Scent: Strong spicy
Uses
Warming to the body
Relieves pain
Helps relieve fatigue
Energizing
Improves digestion

✦ ✦ ✦

Cypress

Cupressus sempervirens
Scent: Woody

Uses

Reduces stress and tension

Relaxes tight muscles

Calming

Promotes restful sleep

Regulates female reproductive system

Reduces perspiration

Helps reduce cellulite deposits

Contracts weak connective tissue

Tones skin

Stops bleeding from injuries

◆ ◆ ◆

Dill

Anethum graveolens
Scent: Spicy

Uses

Reduces stress

Calming

Relieves pain

Promotes restful sleep

Improves digestion

Stimulates lactation in nursing mothers

Repels insects

◆ ◆ ◆

Eucalyptus

Eucalyptus globulus
Scent: Fresh, camphorlike

Uses

Cooling to the body

Relieves pain

Refreshing

Breaks up congestion

Reduces inflammation

Vapors help breathing

Disinfectant

Repels insects

◆ ◆ ◆

Fennel

Foeniculum vulgare
Scent: Strong licorice

Uses

Warming to the body

Relieves pain

Improves digestion

Increases appetite

Contains estrogen-like hormone

Stimulates lactation in nursing mothers

Helps reduce cellulite deposits

Purifying effect on the body

Repels insects

◆ ◆ ◆

Frankincense

Boswellia thurifera
Scent: Woody and camphorlike

Uses

Calming

Helpful for meditation

Promotes restful sleep

Reduces inflammation

Encourages communication

Healing to the skin and wrinkles

✦ ✦ ✦

Geranium

Pelargonium graveolens
Scent: Roselike

Uses

Reduces stress and tension

Calming in small amounts

Stimulating in large amounts

Lessens pain

Mood uplifting

Reduces inflammation

Encourages communication

Helps reduce cellulite deposits

Stops bleeding from injuries

Soothes itching skin

Repels insects

✦ ✦ ✦

Ginger

Zingiber officinale
Scent: Spicy

Uses

Warming to the body

Relaxes tight muscles

Relieves pain

Mood uplifting

Aphrodisiac

Helps relieve fatigue

Energizing

Improves digestion

Increases appetite

Improves mental clarity and memory

✦ ✦ ✦

Grapefruit

Citrus paradisi
Scent: Citrus

Uses

Cooling to the body

Mood uplifting

Helps relieve fatigue

Refreshing

Energizing

Increases physical strength

Improves mental clarity and memory

Helps reduce cellulite deposits

Purifying effect on the body

✦ ✦ ✦

Jasmine

Jasminum officinale
Scent: Sweet floral
Uses
Mood uplifting
Aphrodisiac

◆ ◆ ◆

Juniper Berries

Juniperus communis
Scent: Evergreen forest
Uses
Lessens pain
Energizing
Reduces inflammation
Improves mental clarity and memory
Helps reduce cellulite deposits
Purifying to the body
Soothes insect bites
Repels insects

◆ ◆ ◆

Lavender

Lavandula officinalis
Scent: Fresh and clean
Uses
Reduces stress and tension
Calming in small amounts
Stimulating in large amounts
Relaxes tight muscles
Lessens pain
Promotes restful sleep
Mood uplifting
Balances mood swings
Breaks up congestion
Reduces inflammation
Vapors help breathing
Improves digestion
Purifying to the body
Disinfectant
Healing to the skin
Soothes insect bites
Repels insects

◆ ◆ ◆

Lemon

Citrus limonum

Scent: Lemony

Uses

Cooling to the body

Balancing, calming, or energizing

Balances nervous system

Mood uplifting

Helps relieve fatigue

Refreshing

Improves mental clarity and memory

Helps reduce cellulite deposits

Purifying effect on the body

Stops bleeding from injuries

Disinfectant

Soothes insect bites

✦ ✦ ✦

Lemongrass

Cymbopogon citratus

Scent: Strong lemon

Uses

Calming

Balances nervous system

Mood uplifting

Reduces inflammation

Vapors help breathing

Improves digestion

Stimulates lactation in nursing mothers

Contracts weak connective tissue

Disinfectant

Tones skin

Repels insects

✦ ✦ ✦

Lime

Citrus limetta

Scent: Fresh citrus

Uses

Cooling to the body

Mood uplifting

Helps relieve fatigue

Refreshing

Energizing

Improves mental clarity and memory

Helps reduce cellulite deposits

Purifying effect on the body

Disinfectant

Soothes insect bites

✦ ✦ ✦

Mandarin

Citrus nobilis

Scent: Sweet citrus

Uses

Cooling to the body

Reduces stress and tension

Calming

Mood uplifting

✦ ✦ ✦

Marjoram

Origanum marjorana
Scent: Sweet and spicy
Uses
Warming to the body
Calming
Relaxes tight muscles
Promotes restful sleep
Breaks up congestion
Reduces inflammation
Vapors help breathing
Improves digestion
Disinfectant
Soothes insect bites

✦ ✦ ✦

Melissa

Melissa officinalis
Scent: Lemony
Uses
Reduces stress and anxiety
Calming and relaxing
Relieves aches and pains
Promotes restful sleep
Mood uplifting

✦ ✦ ✦

Myrrh

Commiphora myrrha
Scent: Bitter
Uses
Helpful for meditation
Mood uplifting
Reduces inflammation
Healing to the skin

✦ ✦ ✦

Myrtle

Myrtus communis
Scent: Fresh, camphorlike
Uses
Calming
Vapors help breathing

✦ ✦ ✦

Neroli

Citrus aurantium
Scent: Sweet floral
Uses
Relieves nervous tension
Promotes restful sleep
Mood uplifting

✦ ✦ ✦

Nutmeg

Myristica fragrans
Scent: Spicy
Uses
Calming in small amounts
Stimulating in large amounts
Relaxes tight muscles
Relieves pain
Improves digestion

✦ ✦ ✦

Orange

Citrus aurantium
Scent: Sweet orange
Uses
Cooling to the body
Reduces stress
Calming
Promotes restful sleep
Mood uplifting
Purifying effect on the body

✦ ✦ ✦

Palmarosa

Cymbopogon martini
Scent: Sweet
Uses
Warming to the body
Relaxes tight muscles
Lessens pain
Mood uplifting
Reduces inflammation
Healing, regenerating, moisturizing for skin

✦ ✦ ✦

Patchouli

Pogostemon patchouli
Scent: Musky
Uses
Mood uplifting
Aphrodisiac
Nerve stimulant
Disinfectant
Healing to the skin
Repels insects

✦ ✦ ✦

Black Pepper

Piper nigrum
Scent: Hot and spicy
Uses
Warming to the body
Relaxes tight muscles
Improves digestion

✦ ✦ ✦

Peppermint

Mentha piperita
Scent: Strong mint
Uses
Cooling to the body
Relieves pain
Mood uplifting
Helps relieve fatigue
Aphrodisiac
Refreshing
Energizing
Nerve stimulant
Increases physical strength
Breaks up congestion
Reduces inflammation
Vapors help breathing
Improves digestion
Increases appetite
Reduces lactation in nursing mothers
Improves mental clarity and memory
Soothes itching skin
Repels insects

✦ ✦ ✦

Peru Balsam

Myroxylon pereirae
Scent: Vanilla
Uses
Warming to the body
Calming
Promotes restful sleep
Mood uplifting
Healing to the skin

✦ ✦ ✦

Petitgrain

Citrus bigarade
Scent: Slightly citrus
Uses
Reduces anxiety, stress, and tension
Calming
Promotes restful sleep
Mood uplifting
Improves mental clarity and memory
Healing to the skin

✦ ✦ ✦

Pine

Pinus sylvestris
Scent: Fresh pine
Uses
Lessens pain
Mood uplifting
Helps relieve fatigue
Refreshing
Energizing
Increases physical strength
Breaks up congestion
Vapors help breathing
Improves mental clarity and memory
Purifying effect on the body
Disinfectant

✦ ✦ ✦

Rose

Rosa centifolia
and
Rosa damascena

Scent: Rosy

Uses

Calming

Lessens pain

Mood uplifting

Aphrodisiac

Increases physical strength

Reduces inflammation

Purifying effect on the body

Healing to the skin

✦ ✦ ✦

Rosemary

Rosmarinus officinalis

Scent: Strong camphor

Uses

Relaxes tight muscles

Relieves pain

Mood uplifting

Helps relieve fatigue

Energizing

Nerve stimulant

Vapors help breathing

Improves digestion

Improves mental clarity and memory

Helps reduce cellulite deposits

Purifying effect on the body

Disinfectant

Repels insects

✦ ✦ ✦

Sage

Salvia officinalis

Scent: Spicy

Uses

Lessens pain

Reduces lactation in nursing mothers

Reduces perspiration

Purifying effect on the body

Disinfectant

✦ ✦ ✦

Sandalwood

Santalum album

Scent: Woody

Uses

Reduces stress

Calming

Helpful for meditation

Promotes restful sleep

Mood uplifting

Aphrodisiac

Healing to the skin

✦ ✦ ✦

Spearmint

Mentha spicata
Scent: Minty

Uses

Cooling to the body

Relieves pain

Mood uplifting

Helps relieve fatigue

Aphrodisiac

Refreshing

Energizing

Nerve stimulant

Increases physical strength

Breaks up congestion

Reduces inflammation

Vapors help breathing

Improves digestion

Increases appetite

Improves mental clarity and memory

Soothes itching skin

Repels insects

✦ ✦ ✦

Spruce

Picea mariana
Scent: Sweet pinelike

Uses

Calming

Breaks up congestion

Vapors help breathing

Encourages communication

✦ ✦ ✦

Tea Tree

Melaleuca alternifolia
Scent: Camphorlike

Uses

Lessens pain

Vapors help breathing

Disinfectant

Healing to the skin

✦ ✦ ✦

Thyme

Thymus vulgaris
Scent: Hot and spicy

Uses

Warming to the body

Relaxes tight muscles

Lessens pain

Mood uplifting

Aphrodisiac

Increases physical strength

Breaks up congestion

Reduces inflammation

Vapors help breathing

Improves digestion

Increases appetite

Increases perspiration

Improves mental clarity and memory

Helps reduce cellulite deposits

Purifying effect on the body

Disinfectant

Repels insects

✦ ✦ ✦

Tolu Balsam

Myroxlon toluiferum

Scent: Floral

Uses

Mood uplifting

Fixative for perfumes and fragrances

Deodorant

✦ ✦ ✦

Vetiver

Vetiveria zizanoides

Scent: Earthy

Uses

Reduces stress and tension

Calming

Relaxes tight muscles

Relieves pain

Promotes restful sleep

Increases physical strength

Healing to the skin

Repels insects

✦ ✦ ✦

Ylang-Ylang

Cananga odorata

Scent: Sweet floral

Uses

Calming

Relaxes tight muscles

Lessens pain

Promotes restful sleep

Mood uplifting

Aphrodisiac

Encourages communication

Disinfectant

✦ ✦ ✦

6

QUICK GUIDE TO PROPERTIES

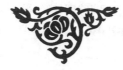

Aphrodisiac   Anise, clary sage, cinnamon, clove, ginger, jasmine, patchouli, peppermint, rose, sandalwood, spearmint, thyme, ylang-ylang

Appetite (*Increases*)   Anise, caraway, chamomile, cinnamon, fennel, ginger, peppermint, spearmint, thyme

Bleeding (*To stop*)   Cypress, geranium, lemon

Breathing   Allspice, anise, (sweet) bay, cajeput, caraway, cedarwood, clove, cubeb, eucalyptus, lavender, lemongrass, marjoram, myrtle, peppermint, pine, rosemary, spearmint, spruce, tea tree, thyme

Calming   Allspice, anise, (sweet) basil, (sweet) bay, benzoin, bois de rose, cajeput, cedarwood, celery, chamomile, clary sage, cypress, dill, frankincense, geranium, lavender, lemon, lemongrass, mandarin, marjoram, melissa, myrtle, nutmeg, orange, Peru balsam, petitgrain, rose, sandalwood, spruce, vetiver, ylang-ylang

Cellulite   (Sweet) basil, benzoin, celery, cinnamon, cypress, fennel, geranium, grapefruit, juniper berries, lemon, lime, rosemary, thyme

Communication (*Encourages*)   Clary sage, frankincense, geranium, spruce, ylang-ylang

Congestion   Benzoin, cajeput, cubeb, eucalyptus, lavender, marjoram, peppermint, pine, spearmint, spruce, thyme

Connective Tissue (*Tightens*)   Cypress, lemongrass

Cooling Eucalyptus, grapefruit, lemon, lime, mandarin, orange, peppermint, spearmint

Digestion Allspice, anise, (sweet) basil, (sweet) bay, caraway, cardamom, chamomile, cinnamon, clary sage, clove, coriander, cubeb, cumin, dill, fennel, ginger, lavender, lemongrass, marjoram, nutmeg, black pepper, peppermint, rosemary, spearmint, thyme

Disinfectant Allspice, (sweet) bay, bergamot, cajeput, cinnamon, clove, eucalyptus, lavender, lemon, lemongrass, lime, marjoram, patchouli, pine, rosemary, sage, tea tree, thyme, ylang-ylang

Energizing Cumin, ginger, grapefruit, juniper berries, lemon, lime, peppermint, pine, rosemary, spearmint

Fatigue (*Relieves*) (Sweet) basil, bergamot, cinnamon, clove, coriander, cumin, ginger, grapefruit, lemon, lime, peppermint, pine, rosemary, spearmint

Female Reproductive System Regulator Clary sage, cypress, fennel

Fixative Benzoin, patchouli, sandalwood, tolu balsam

Inflammation Benzoin, chamomile, eucalyptus, frankincense, geranium, juniper berries, lavender, lemongrass, marjoram, myrrh, palmarosa, peppermint, rose, spearmint, thyme

Insect Bites (Sweet) basil, chamomile, juniper berries, lavender, lemon, lime, marjoram

Insect Repellent (Sweet) bay, cajeput, cedarwood, cinnamon, clove, dill, eucalyptus, fennel, geranium, lavender, lemongrass, patchouli, peppermint, rosemary, spearmint, thyme, vetiver

Lactation (*To decrease*) Peppermint, sage   (*To increase*) Anise, (sweet) basil, caraway, dill, fennel, lemongrass

Meditation Benzoin, cedarwood, frankincense, myrrh, sandalwood

Mental Clarity and Memory Improvement (Sweet) basil, (sweet) bay, cardamom, clove, coriander, ginger, grapefruit, juniper berries, lemon, lime, peppermint, petitgrain, rosemary, spearmint, thyme

Moisturizing Aloe, bois de rose, palmarosa

Mood Swings Lavender

Mood Uplifting Allspice, (sweet) basil, benzoin, bergamot, bois de rose, cardamom, cinnamon, clove, geranium, ginger, grapefruit, jasmine, lavender, lemon, lemongrass, lime, mandarin, melissa, myrrh, neroli, orange, palmarosa, patchouli, peppermint, Peru balsam, petitgrain, pine, rose, rosemary, sandalwood, spearmint, thyme, tolu balsam, ylang-ylang

Muscle Tension Relief Allspice, (sweet) bay, benzoin, cajeput, cedarwood, cinnamon, cypress, ginger, lavender, nutmeg, palmarosa, black pepper, rosemary, thyme, vetiver

Nerve Stimulant Patchouli, peppermint, rosemary, spearmint

Nervous System (*Balancing*) Bergamot, lemon, lemongrass

Pain Allspice, anise, (sweet) basil, (sweet) bay, bois de rose, cajeput, caraway, cardamom, cedarwood, chamomile, cinnamon, clary sage, clove, coriander, cubeb, cumin, dill, eucalyptus, fennel, geranium, ginger, juniper berries, lavender, melissa, nutmeg, palmarosa, peppermint, pine, rose, rosemary, sage, spearmint, tea tree, thyme, vetiver, ylang-ylang

Physical Endurance Grapefruit, peppermint, pine, rose, spearmint, thyme, vetiver

Perspiration (*Increases*) (Sweet) bay, thyme   (*Reduces*) Cypress, sage

Purifying (Sweet) basil, celery, fennel, grapefruit, juniper berries, lavender, lemon, lime, orange, pine, rose, rosemary, sage, thyme

Refreshing Eucalyptus, grapefruit, lemon, lime, peppermint, pine, spearmint

Skin Care Aloe, benzoin, bois de rose, chamomile, frankincense, lavender, myrrh, palmarosa, patchouli, Peru balsam, petitgrain, rose, sandalwood, tea tree, vetiver

Skin (*Stops itching*) Geranium, peppermint, Peru balsam, spearmint

Skin Toning Cypress, lemongrass

Sleep Restfully Allspice, anise, (sweet) basil, (sweet) bay, benzoin, bois de rose, cajeput, cedarwood, celery, chamomile, clary sage, cypress, dill, frankincense, lavender, marjoram, melissa, neroli, orange, Peru balsam, petitgrain, sandalwood, vetiver, ylang-ylang

Stress Relief Allspice, benzoin, bergamot, bois de rose, cedarwood, celery, chamomile, clary sage, cypress, dill, geranium, lavender, mandarin, melissa, orange, petitgrain, sandalwood, vetiver

Warming Allspice, benzoin, cajeput, cardamom, cinnamon, clove, cumin, fennel, ginger, marjoram, palmarosa, black pepper, Peru balsam, thyme

About the Authors

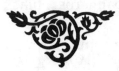

Carol Schiller and David Schiller have been working with formulating aromatherapy blends since 1986. Their aromatherapy articles have appeared in the following magazines: *Mothering, Massage, Health World, Herb Quarterly,* and *Your Health.* They also instruct classes for colleges and hold training courses for companies.

INDEX

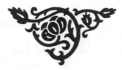